That Silver-Haired Daddy of Mine:

Family Caregiving With a Nurse Care-Manager Approach

Based on the *Your Support Nurse* service,

tested nationwide

Daniel R. Tobin, M.D.
With
Karen Lindsey

AuthorHouse™
1663 Liberty Drive, Suite 200
Bloomington, IN 47403
www.authorhouse.com
Phone: 1-800-839-8640

© 2008 Daniel R. Tobin, M.D. with Karen Lindsey. All rights reserved.

No part of this book may be reproduced, stored in a retrieval system, or transmitted by any means without the written permission of the author.

First published by AuthorHouse 9/30/2008

ISBN: 978-1-4389-0439-9 (sc)

Library of Congress Control Number: 2008908884

Printed in the United States of America
Bloomington, Indiana

This book is printed on acid-free paper.

Dedication

This book is dedicated to Richard Liebich for his unwavering support and mentorship in building sustainable services for people with serious illnesses. In his daily work he continues to create positive change, utilizing critical thinking, perseverance, and outcomes-based, high-engagement philanthropy.

Contents

Introduction	xiii
Chapter 1 – A Care-Manager Approach to Healthcare	1
Chapter 2 – Coordinating Your Aging Parent's Needs	19
Chapter 3 – Physician Support and Health Literacy	41
Chapter 4 – Information Support and Coordinating Care	59
Chapter 5 – Guidance and Emotional Support	75
Chapter 6 – Tangible Support and Extended Planning	89
Appendix – Resources for Caregivers	115
References	121
About Your Support Nurse	125

Acknowledgements

Thanks to everyone who has supported the theory that patients and family caregivers facing advancing illness can significantly benefit from routine, good quality care coordination, and health counseling.

Special thanks to all the healthcare practitioners and leaders who contributed to the programs we have been involved with over the years.

Thanks to everyone within the VA Healthcare Network Upstate New York who helped me get started in the field of heath counseling. Special thanks to Linda Weiss, Paula Hemmings, Bill Gorman, and Fred Malphurs.

Thanks to Dale Larson, Joe Odonnell, Richard Dellepenna, Perry Fine, Sylvia McSkimmings, Ira Byock, Kathy Foley, Myra Christopher, and Jian Gao. Special thanks to Elinor Ginzler for being there for me over the years.

Special thanks to Drea Foster for being a part of our team.

Thanks to Pam Georgiana, Sandy Aldrich, and everyone at Borders who have helped focus attention on family caregiving. Special thanks to Ken Armstrong for opening up opportunities for me to contribute in the field of caregiving.

Thanks to Catherine Heslep, Dave Shotwell, Amy Silverstein Levner, Suzanne Lutz, Jane Lincoln, Eugene Scanzera, and everyone at AARP who have made family caregiving a part of their agenda. Special thanks to Bill Novelli, who has supported innovative family caregiving, care coordination, and health counseling for many years.

Thanks to Blake Martin, Angel Carl, Brian Petranick, and everyone at Right At Home for their support and collaboration. Special thanks to Allen Hager for his vision, leadership, and evolving friendship.

Thanks to Ed Ruckle for directing our media strategy. Special thanks to Tom Wilson for his guidance and being a mentor in advertising strategy and development. Thanks to Sam Smith, Judy Painter, and everyone at PainterSmith for their invaluable creative contributions.

A special note of gratitude to Beth Liebich, who helped build the Center for Advanced Illness Coordinated Care, for being a guiding light to this work. Thanks to everyone at the Charitable Leadership Foundation who has helped support our efforts and Care Support of America. Thanks to everyone at Care Support of America for their dedication and hard work and for helping to see the wish fulfilled. Thanks to all the nurse care managers who are using this model every day. Special thanks to

Jeremy Nicholson for his direct contribution to the content and organization of this book, to Rick Gleber for all the hard work and collaboration in bringing this work to the public, and to Joe Englehardt, who has supported this vision from its inception, helped create the research to develop it, and developed many of the concepts in this book.

Thanks to Marnie Cochran for her guidance in planning this book. Thanks to Jo Ann Lenney for her talented help with editing the manuscript.

It is a privilege to have, once again, worked with Karen Lindsey to create a book that can help others help themselves. Her talents and focus on the integrity of communication are evident throughout this entire work.

To Robin, Brian, and Jeremy, my wonderful wife and children, who supported and participated in the creative pursuit of blazing new trails.

Introduction

The excitement in the room was palpable as we made the decision. After years of work, we were going to bring our care-manager services directly to the consumer. The services had now proven to have positive results for family caregivers and patients facing serious illness. We were ready.

Eight years earlier we had begun our work in a Veteran's Administration (VA) medical center in Albany, New York, with one simple concept: routine healthcare needed to practically and emotionally support family caregivers and patients facing advanced chronic illness. We formed an organization that we called the Coordinated Care Group, which later changed its name to Care Support of America (CSA). There were six of us then (later we would expand to about 20). We knew that a focus on the whole person and the needs of the patient and family, rather than simply the symptoms or disease, aided clinical care and well-being.

Crucial to our goal was the idea that we create a form of nurse care-manager service that would be directly accessible to anyone who needed it, anywhere in the country. The issue of baby boomers caregiving for aging parents had become a public and painful topic. Newspaper articles and TV features frequently addressed the needs that family caregivers were experiencing daily as they tended to their parents. We saw the limits of what was provided to the elderly ill. Medicare, for example, though it paid for senior healthcare, did not underwrite the counseling necessary to help most family caregivers to coordinate meeting their parents' needs. Nor did most commercial health-insurance plans. Yet we also knew that much could be done if caregivers were only offered the right information and taught the right skills. This book is a part of our efforts to bring valuable information to as many of these people as possible.

Our version of care coordination and health counseling, which is outlined in this book, involves a practical approach to coordinating aging parents' care that has both short- and long-term results. We have defined eight activities that instruct family caregivers, along with their parents who become patients. First we emphasize family caregiving. Then we spell out how to understand chronic illness and to coordinate care. Though attending to medical needs is in the hands of the physician, knowing what questions to ask that physician is enormously important. Second we address the practical and emotional aspect of caring for your aging parent's needs, which comprise more than merely the medical. The elements that we'll outline in this book will provide a framework to help you organize your thinking about the diverse needs that come with your parent's chronic and serious illness. Within this framework, you will be provided with methods of gathering information about the illness, strategies for talking with the physicians, ways of clarifying treatment options, and techniques for bridging the gap between medical and nonmedical home care.

In addition, elements of our program can help family caregivers and patients to cope with illness by recognizing and defining their emotional reactions. We offer strategies for seeking assistance within the family and the community, and we provide problem-solving approaches to self-management issues as they arise. Finally we present elements designed to help you prepare for the potential worsening of your parent's illness—to learn the possible course of the disease and discuss planning with the physicians about how to deal with each likely stage of its progression.

As we sat around our conference table outlining this book, we talked about what we had seen family caregivers and their parents face over and over again. We knew that physicians, hospital systems, assisted-living facilities, nursing homes, and managed-care insurers were hampered by the fact that care coordination and practical support that bridged medical and nonmedical home care were not routinely or consistently built into current care delivery. Studies had shown that despite all the services available within healthcare, many people remained confused and unable to work their way through the system. The need for more accessible care managers to address patients' and caregivers' concerns had been well documented, but comprehensive solutions to the problem were not yet evident within most care-delivery systems. We knew that a focus on the whole person and the needs of the patient and family was necessary. We realized that there were 30 million baby-boomer caregivers, 7 million of whom lived more than 400 miles from their parents, who were facing the daily struggle of understanding and planning for their parents' needs.

We began our experimental program by integrating nurses or social workers into the system to act as care coordinators for patients and caregivers, providing information, planning modes of assistance, and offering emotional support. We studied the positive effects of these services and were supported by the leadership of VA Healthcare Upstate New York, who saw the human as well as the economic value in our work.

Two years later, we developed a training center that has since helped to implement nationwide quality-improvement programs and services in advanced-illness coordinated care outside of the VA healthcare system. We gathered a diverse health-services research group to study the programs we implemented, and we further refined our work and explored additional ways to implement it. This group included nurses, nurse practitioners, psychologists, gerontologists, chaplains, primary and specialty physicians and pain specialists, and social workers, all focused on creating a nurse care-manager model that would be comprehensive, reproducible, and flexible.

In implementing these programs over the years, we noticed specific areas of care that could be improved with more information and guidance. We trained our nurses and social workers to help family caregivers and patients address both their fears and the practical and emotional issues that arise when dealing with a chronic and advancing illness. We focused on creating individual care coordination and health-counseling plans based on the unique nature of each family situation and individual decision-making style. We found ways to promote shared decision making in helping patients and families to understand their doctors and communicate with them. We saw that a loved one's illness often affects a large network of family and friends who are involved in day-to-day care, as well as the primary caregiver. Therefore we decided that our program had to incorporate such an extended network.

We also found that many patients didn't fully understand their illness—nor did their family caregivers. Using a technique known as structured conversation, we helped people learn to stay in control of their situation, make informed decisions, and remain empowered even in difficult circumstances. Therefore, in order to truly help family caregivers and their ill parents, we found that we also had to incorporate and support their extended network of caregivers.

Our care-coordination support has been specifically created to work with the treating physician's goals and help patients and families cope with difficult situations that arise. We have seen that while there are some parts of dealing with such serious illness that are unavoidably and permanently difficult, there are many other problems that are easily minimized or entirely preventable with a little information, planning, and support. Basically, we have learned that practical, short-term interventions in a few key areas can make a tremendous difference in people's lives. For example, our group devised a simple five-question form to guide patient-physician communication and help alleviate patients' uncertainty around diagnosis, treatment, and prognosis. This brief form greatly helped patients and their caregivers better understand the treatment that they were receiving, communicate more effectively with their doctors, and more easily plan for future needs. These improvements in information, communication, and planning helped caregivers and their parents feel more at ease, more in control, and better able to cope with the illness. All of these benefits came from one brief form containing a few key questions.

Over the years, we saw that a single nurse care manager was able to accomplish a great deal of care coordination and guidance for family members in a short time. Being able to help normalize the situation by explaining to family caregivers some of the basics involved in navigating complex healthcare circumstances (often including finding credible private-duty, in-home providers) resulted in immediate relief.

In the years since then, we have piloted and implemented our care-manager programs within large group health systems like Kaiser Permanente; major plans like Blue Cross Blue Shield of Massachusetts, Montana, Northeast and Northwestern New York;

Medicare HMOs like Oxford Health Care and Humana; in Catholic Healthcare Hospital systems, and in nursing homes throughout the country. Family caregiving as a community issue is also being increasingly recognized in the workplace. These programs are just some of the current attempts to recognize the value of comprehensive care coordination and support within hospital and managed Medicare systems.

Most doctor's offices, hospitals, and insurance settings still offer no comprehensive, ongoing care coordination and support services as part of routine care. However, within such systems and settings, we were funded to do millions of dollars of research, and we have proven that our program of care has been developed and tested, and that a care-manager approach works well to improve the quality of life for family caregivers and their parents. Despite these successes in our ability to improve the lives and care of family caregivers and patients, our attempts to expand our care-manager approach into regular physician office practices have not yet resulted in a reimbursement model for family caregiving, health counseling, and care coordination.

So we decided to write this book in the hope that it will help people nationwide who do not as yet have all their needs met by their healthcare services as they are currently delivered. We had to figure out ways to get our particular approach to people who needed it. This book, much like a road map, is one of the ways we are bringing our guidance and support to you. We hope that it will inspire public awareness and demand, as well as providing immediate aid to people who are unable to locate or access personal care managers. The eight activities you will discover in this book are not meant to be a panacea; nor are they meant to be all-encompassing. Rather they comprise a basic framework to support the care and direction you will receive from your doctor. We hope that you find this framework helpful and that you experience the same improvements in control, efficacy, decision making, and well-being that we have been able to bring to others throughout our continued efforts.

Though I have done the actual work of shaping and writing this book, the material, as you see in this introduction, was provided by the staff of Care Support of America. It is their work as well as mine. It is also the work of Joe Englehardt, Ph.D., who has been a creative collaborator in the development of this model. Further, he has led research to support it and has helped shape the activities and concepts throughout this book.

Chapter 1 –
A Care-Manager Approach to Healthcare

At 58, Jessica Austen[1] is a comfortably successful writer in Los Angeles. Her life changed drastically when her father was diagnosed with colon cancer several years ago. Soon the cancer spread, and Mr. Austen, 88, has grown increasingly fragile. His chief caregiver has been Jessica's mother, now 90. She is caring for him in the home they have lived in for most of their married life. It's a lovely home, but it's in Washington, D.C., far away from Jessica and her three brothers. The four of them are paying for private-duty, in-home care services to help Mrs. Austen care for her husband, now bedridden, and their home. Jessica is close to both her parents, and she flies cross-country once a month to help them coordinate doctor's visits and laboratory tests. She also helps with their home-care requirements, with organizing medication, paying bills, and keeping track of daily household needs. Jessica's

---

[1] This and all other patient names are invented, to protect privacy. In some cases, we have used composites of several patients in order to economically illustrate a point.

brothers call her, each other, and their parents often, but they are rarely willing or able to fly to Washington and help personally. Jessica is growing increasingly stressed. She sees her mother becoming emotionally as well as physically exhausted. Jessica and her parents have begun discussing the possibility of their moving into an assisted-living or nursing home, but it isn't easy. They are overwhelmed by the thought of leaving their beloved home and of losing their independence. If he were to go to a nursing home, they would lose even their life together. Jessica finds herself feeling guilty. Is she doing enough to help her parents? How can she be sure that the private-duty, in-home care services are thorough enough and that the aides are really trustworthy?

Dave Leonard is a 49-year-old attorney living in St. Louis. He is the only child of his widowed 82-year-old father, who has both uncontrolled diabetes and advancing heart disease. Mr. Leonard was recently admitted to the hospital for the fifth time in one year. Dave travels to Oshkosh to visit his father every six or eight weeks, and is increasingly concerned about whether Mr. Leonard can continue living at home safely. Mrs. Leonard died two years ago from a heart attack, and while several local friends look in on Mr. Leonard from time to time, the hospital social worker has strongly recommended that he consider getting daily help at home or move to a more secure environment. Intensely independent, Mr. Leonard explains to his son that he cannot afford any of the services that are recommended. Dave was never close to his father, but he feels a responsibility to be with him as often as possible. He has considered moving Mr. Leonard into his home, but his wife is already overwhelmed by the job of raising their children and doesn't want that. As Mr. Leonard's condition deteriorates, Dave feels frustrated and confused.

Barb Orion lives in Philadelphia, a few blocks away from the assisted-living home her 85-year-old mother lives in. This saves Barb the extensive traveling that people like Jessica and Dave face, but creates its own set of problems. Mrs. Orion constantly pressures Barb to visit her for dinner and help her get about town. Mrs. Orion has early Alzheimer's, and cannot understand that Barb's high-level executive job keeps her busy. All Mrs. Orion can see is that Barb's two children are in college and that this could free up time for Barb to spend with her. Barb's commitment to her work, she complains, is selfish. Mrs. Orion had always been an aloof mother, but her dementia has created personality changes that Barb finds difficult and sometimes frightening. She wants to be a good daughter and do whatever she can for her mother, but she is increasingly upset by the inroads Mrs. Orion's demands are making in her life.

Mrs. Orion also has heart disease, and the doctors are suggesting open-heart surgery. This will force Barb into an even greater caregiving role. Meanwhile her mother is increasingly hostile toward her. "You were never a good daughter," Mrs. Orion screams. This is untrue and Barb knows it, but it always hits a nerve. How far should a middle-aged woman go to be a "good daughter" to a mother toward whom she has always felt ambivalent, and whose dementia has turned her into someone hostile and alienating?

Jessica, Dave, and Barb are all baby boomers who find themselves caught in the daily struggles and stress of caregiving for their aging parents. Though the specifics of their situations are different, all three are having trouble understanding how to gain control of managing their parents' illnesses. They foresee years of involvement in their parents' care, and all of them want to do the best they can.

They are not alone. There are 30 million baby boomers caring for their parents, 7 million of whom are long-distance caregivers. Research shows both an objective and subjective burden in caring for parents with advanced illness (Montgomery, Gonyea, & Hooyman, 1985). Baby boomers in this role have increased risk of both physical and emotional problems. The parents too have difficulty with the role reversal that has been imposed on them. They often expect that their children will help them, but they do not want to be a burden. The emotions between aging parents and their adult children are many and intense, carrying all the love and all the anger of half a century or more. As the parents' illnesses progress, both they and their children experience a sense of loss of control. Part of this is the result of the disease itself, along with its relentless reminder of mortality. Medicine can do much to alleviate suffering and often to prolong life, but finally the aging body wears down.

Another part of the loss, however, is the complexity and strangeness of healthcare particulars. Caregivers have to deal with the medical world, legal concerns, financial issues, other family responsibilities, housekeeping, different needs, and disparate institutions. Though no one can prevent illness and, eventually, death, the chaos surrounding the process is a different story. It doesn't need to be this hard. Reproducible solutions are unfolding by which professionals can work with each struggling family. There are a number of organizations that are working on this, including my own, Care Support of America (CSA). It is out of my work in this organization that this book has arisen.

Central to my work is the concept of the "care manager," a trained nurse or social worker who helps a family coordinate all the aspects of caring for a seriously ill person. Later in this chapter, you'll find a discussion of the origin and role of the care manager. But before that, I want to backtrack a little—to explain the genesis of my work.

Ten years ago, I began working at a Veterans Administration (VA) medical center, helping patients and family members facing advancing illness and coping with end-of-life situations. I saw many struggles that caregivers and patients were facing on both practical and emotional levels. I also noticed that there were basic needs of family caregivers and patients that could be met if information and guidance was standardized. Some doctors did a great job of spending time with family caregivers and patients to explain the many parts of coordinating care, but more time was needed to help them understand and organize home care and the practical as well as emotional aspects of advancing chronic illness. The doctor's office had a great opportunity to provide care coordination and health counseling, but few had a standardized way to deliver these services. Yet there was clearly a need for this—a road map that would help family caregivers and patients understand the terrain in front of them. Virtually every patient I worked with needed this on an ongoing basis, but it was hard to find it. Visiting nurses as part of what is called certified home care, hospital discharge planners, hospital case managers, and others do provide excellent coordination, but too often for only brief periods of time.

Many physicians believe that poor coordination of care generally leads to unnecessary hospitalizations, nursing-home placements, and diagnostic tests (Partnership for Solutions, 2004). In a Chronic Illness Physicians Survey conducted by Mathematica Policy Research in 2001, 66 percent of physicians surveyed indicated that their training did not prepare them to coordinate in-home and community services.

So I decided to develop a model to help guide patients and their families through some of the processes of facing illness and eventual death. Central to this model was that care managers would be available directly to the customer: the organization would be exclusively for this purpose. One phone call would be all a customer would need to be given information and to hire a care manager. This direct accessibility would put the customer in control of the process, with no third party involved.

This process involved medical issues, but equally important, the range of practical, psychological, and personal concerns that inevitably accompany coping with long-term illness. I had a sense of the care coordination and health counseling that could be helpful and I was determined to figure out a way to make it operational. In 1999, I wrote a book about this model based on my experiences at the VA medical center (Tobin, 1999).

One thing I had noticed at the VA medical center was that most of the patients had visits from family members—often frequent visits. I saw all the difficulty these people faced, wanting to help their loved ones, and how much responsibility they had to deal with beyond the physical needs that the hospital staff provided for. Often, in fact, my work had involved the family as much as the patient.

As I looked around for ways to help, I discovered the work the prestigious Institute of Medicine had done in 1997. They outlined four domains of care that would be helpful for all patients and family caregivers to address: the physical, practical, emotional, and spiritual. Clearly physicians tend to the physical, but often the practical, emotional, and spiritual issues are delegated to other healthcare providers or ancillary staff—or to no one at all. It is in these areas that a care manager can be extremely helpful.

The more I read and observed, the more I realized the importance of helping families create individualized plans of ongoing care at home. Often getting only a few hours of private-duty, in-home care could, along with an action plan that was coordinated with the physician's office, help seniors be safe at home for many months instead of having to move to nursing homes.

Though the overall structure of all the plans should be the same, it was important to honor the different needs of the diverse people involved. Everyone had to be clear on understanding their physicians' treatment plans, but the variables of each caregiver's life and decision-making style were equally important. Without addressing both fears and practical issues, patients and family members would struggle with a sense of chaos in dealing with advancing illness. Nor could we assume that the families *did* understand the doctors' treatment plans. Even with the most attentive doctor explaining things to them, many family members (and patients) don't understand fully what they are told. But they often nod politely while the doctor talks to them, afraid to appear either rude or ignorant.

As I observed the response of patients and family caregivers when they were facing advancing illness, I decided that there really were ways to help them gain control of their situations. I created a mode of structured conversations in which I sat with the patient and/or family members and asked specific, standardized questions. First I asked what *their* questions were. Where had they gone to address each of these, and did they get the information they needed? What did the patient and each family member fear?

There was never a universal answer, or even uniform questions from them. Each family had its own specific concerns, determined by the nature of the illness, the family dynamics over the years, and the particular lives lived by each family member. These conversations didn't take a long time. It became crystal clear to me that with only a small amount of standardized information and guidance, we could help these people improve the patient's care and the quality of all their lives.

I realized too that a great deal of assistance could be given in a relatively short period of time. This was exciting. I began to recognize that this had implications beyond the VA setting. I could expand the structured conversations that I was using to be helpful in many different contexts. The practical aspect of coping with illness would involve helping patients and family members coordinate care. But there was more. I was fascinated by the different ways that emotional and spiritual coping could occur. I wanted to understand what characteristics and strengths helped certain people cope better than others. I found also that many people questioned the meaning of their lives when they had to face their own or a loved one's advancing illness.

In 2000, I was given an opportunity to further expand the work I'd begun, when I was hired as a consultant by VA Healthcare Network Upstate New York. My job involved training nurses and social workers in the kind of structured conversations I had used with patients. They would then be able to facilitate both care coordination and therapeutic health counseling for patients facing advancing illness and for their family members.

It was at this juncture that I spent time reflecting on my life's experiences, both personal and clinical, in order to create a practical short-term model of care that could help patients and families cope with serious illness and find a positive, proactive approach to aging. I wanted the work to be based on proven health counseling and to combine a "street smart" approach with clinical excellence. I drew on years of working different jobs as a waiter, restaurant manager, general physician, eye surgeon, health counselor, and palliative-care physician. Combining the practical nature of a surgeon and the listening skills of a counselor, condensing 10 years of psychodynamic psychotherapy that I underwent from ages 25 through 35, I then created an advanced-illness coordinated-care model. I felt I knew how to teach the skills of a standardized model that could meet patients and their families where they were in life and appreciate the practical, emotional, and spiritual aspects of coping with illness.

This advanced-illness coordinated-care work, which had begun in five VA medical centers, grew into training programs for over 500 nurses and social workers throughout the country in progressive hospital systems, nursing homes, and a few specific managed Medicare settings. It became obvious that I could no longer do this training on my own. Two people in particular were of enormous help in those early days. I was joined by Dale Larson, Ph.D., a professor of Counseling Psychology at Santa Clara University. A pioneer in merging health psychology within the American hospice movement's development, he immediately understood the value of the interface of advanced-illness health counseling and routine care.

The other was Joe Engelhardt, Ph.D., a social worker and health services researcher who helped expand the earlier model of care coordination and health counseling. Through his work, we got grants for five major studies, including two with Medicare programs. The studies all showed that the process could significantly improve the quality of life for patients and their caregivers. One of the most dramatic results was a decrease in unnecessary hospitalizations. Social workers and nurses worked with family caregivers and patients. The caregivers no longer had to spend hours in a hit-or-miss search for information about each new issue that came up—medical, legal, or emotional. Freed from the frenzy of the search, caregivers found the quality of their care, and of their lives, improved significantly.

As we expanded our care-manager model within hospitals and Medicare health maintenance organizations (HMOs), it became apparent that our methods were successful among much larger populations than our earlier work had suggested. Unfortunately, it was also apparent that neither Medicare nor commercial insurance companies would be able to pay for family caregiver care-manager services in the foreseeable future.

We would clearly have to create a model that would be at least reasonably affordable. Luckily, "we" had now grown to include several others—nurses, chaplains, even a doctor or two.

In 2002, I was fortunate enough to meet a local philanthropist who would begin to teach me the rigors of business and entrepreneurship. Using what I learned from him, and with the guidance of a small board of directors, I created a nonprofit organization called the Center for Advanced Illness Coordinated Care (CAICC). Then, in 2004, I formed Care Support of America (CSA) as a for-profit corporation. And, in 2006, CSA added a program called Your Support Nurse, offering care-manager services directly to the consumer.

Your Support Nurse tested well in market research and showed that long-distance as well as local baby boomers would purchase an affordable, proven, and practical service to help them become more effective family caregivers. "The sandwich generation"—the generation of adult children who are baby boomers simultaneously taking care of their parents and their own children—told us that it would take a shift for consumers to purchase a healthcare service that was not covered by either their parents' Medicare insurance or their own health insurance. It would be a serious effort, but we were determined to create the marketing plan and advertising materials to demonstrate that quality help is available for overwhelmed family caregivers, in the form of a nurse care manager. We chose a nurse as our care-manager model, as the nurses we trained were comfortable with advancing illness and were interested in bringing their experience to our program.

What Is a Care Manager?

Though CSA's approach to care management is unique, the concept of a "care manager" isn't. In fact, it isn't even new.

A care manager is a health professional, usually a nurse or a social worker, who helps people find and organize services in every area they are needed. A care manager can help people coordinate and activate resources like home healthcare, durable medical equipment, and transportation to doctor's visits. They can help in the decision making and logistics for patients who need or wish to relocate to assisted living.

The Unique Needs of Chronic Illness Care

Healthcare delivery falls into two broad categories: acute and chronic. Acute medical care is needed for rapid-onset, time-limited health problems: a broken bone, an infection, a first heart attack. The term suggests an intense problem that is expected to respond to treatment in a short time.

Chronic care, on the other hand, is needed for diseases that last for a long time and worsen periodically—heart disease, high blood pressure, lung disease, Alzheimer's—or for the inevitable frailty that usually comes with living for a very long time. In contrast to acute care, chronic care may require long and ongoing periods of assistance, usually lasting for the balance of the patient's lifetime. It is this chronic disease care that this book focuses on.

Sometimes, an acute disease becomes chronic: when a first heart attack becomes chronic congestive heart failure, for example, or when cancer spreads and metastasizes. Chronic illness may or may not require caregiving: asthma, diabetes, or arthritis may be sporadically disabling, but are controllable to the extent that the patient's daily life isn't impaired. When chronic illness involves daily limitation of movement, it is called *serious chronic illness*. And when serious chronic illness becomes progressive and nonreversible, it is called *advanced illness*.

From the time serious chronic illness begins, there are usually a multitude of physical, practical, and emotional issues to be faced. Many seniors, often managing multiple chronic illnesses, may see an average of almost 15 doctors a year and fill an average of 50 prescriptions (Partnership for Solutions, 2004).

Almost half of all Americans, from all parts of our society, are living with chronic health conditions. Predictably, many of them need a lot of care. In 2001, care provided to people with chronic conditions accounted for 83 percent of healthcare spending (Partnership for Solutions, 2004). Technological advances in medicine have increased life spans, and we are seeing more and more of the chronic diseases associated with advanced age. New heart medications help chronic congestive heart failure patients do much better for longer periods of time, and the latest treatments for cancer are keeping the chronic nature of some incurable cancers under control for many years.

Hence many doctors and medical researchers have focused their attention on the care of patients with ongoing disease. Research has found that, for the most part, the behavior of doctors, more than of anyone else, has the greatest impact on health outcomes in acute care. For example, in acute illnesses, only a surgeon can mend a complex broken bone and only a doctor can prescribe the correct medication for an infection. The most important factor in a good outcome is the accuracy of the diagnosis and the effectiveness of the treatments.

In contrast, with chronic disease it is usually the behaviors of patients and families that have the greatest impact on health outcomes. For example, an Alzheimer's patient living at home, unable to care for himself, needs to take his prescribed medications. The caregiver's ability to manage the medication regimen is crucial. Similarly a patient with advanced metastatic cancer becomes physically unable to care for herself, and she may become incontinent. The family caregiver must be able to bathe the patient, bring her the bedpan, and sometimes change her diapers, although later in the course of illness the family may have a health aide who will do those things.

Given this perspective, to achieve the most effective outcomes for people, it would make sense that care delivery would be molded around the factor (doctor's behavior or patient/family behavior) that is most likely to improve the outcomes. Almost everyone has experienced the way care delivery in acute medicine is shaped around doctors' schedules. The most common example can be found in the doctors' waiting rooms. Although extended waits may be difficult for the patients, it is clearly the most convenient way to organize the doctors' time and deliver care to all the patients. Logic would then suggest that care delivery should be shaped around patients in chronic care situations. For example, if a specialized diet does not take into account the patient's aversion to certain foods, she may refuse the diet altogether.

As the condition worsens, more and more areas of concern arise, and one or two caregivers, even with the support of friends, can become overwhelmed. Just as the doctor needs other specialists such as consultants and nurses as assistants, so the caregivers need further support. A care-manager approach is the template of this support.

Following are some examples of where a care-manager approach can be helpful:

- If you feel unfamiliar with the disease(s) that your loved one has been diagnosed with and you want to be sure all your questions are answered to your satisfaction no matter how complicated the subject matter may be.

- If you are unsure which caregiving problems you should address first.

- If you want coaching on what to ask the doctor and how to ask it in a way that gives you the clearest and most complete answers.

- If you feel you are doing all the caregiving you can and still don't feel things are going as you would like.

- If you want to be sure you are getting the most value for your healthcare dollar.

- If you don't know where to begin in solving caregiving problems.

- If you want to know if the caregiving job you are doing is a good one.

Care-manager services can save you a great deal of money by reducing travel expenses, lessening unnecessary hospitalizations, and coordinating care with you in an efficient and productive manner. Further, a professional care manager can help alleviate the emotional stress of navigating complex unfamiliar medical and nonmedical situations with information and guidance.

CSA's nurse care-manager program has been proven able to bridge the medical and nonmedical care that patients receive by working with them and their family caregivers on the phone or in the parents' home, as well as with a local nurse who is able to assess home safety and the well-being of the senior. A nurse care manager experienced in serious chronic illness can work with the doctor's office to get helpful information as well as improve communication with the office. This reduces the time that the doctor must spend explaining specific facts and issues, which can lead to responding better to patients and family caregivers.

Your Support Nurse care-manager service has been successfully launched throughout the country because of the response to the internet presence at yoursupportnurse.com. The eight activities outlined throughout this book will give you specific questions and action steps in our nurse care-manager approach to solve caregiving problems.

Chapter 2 –
Coordinating Your Aging Parent's Needs

What Are You Facing?

Many family caregivers slip into the role of caregiving without thinking of it in such terms. As a parent develops serious chronic illness, with expanding needs for care, both parent and caregiver often feel overwhelmed. Added to this, the fact that our country's healthcare system is set up to provide temporary acute, rather than continuous, care creates a difficult situation. The system is both understaffed and fragmented, unable to completely handle the needs of people with serious chronic illness or of their caregivers (Institute of Medicine, 2001). Patients with chronic conditions often receive conflicting advice and even conflicting diagnoses from different physicians. Drug-to-drug interactions are also common, sometimes resulting in hospitalization and, infrequently, death (Partnership for Solutions, 2004). In fact, the Institute of Medicine concluded: "Our current method of organizing and delivering care is unable to meet the expectations of patients and their families because the science and technologies involved in health care—the knowledge, skills, care interventions, devices, and drugs—have advanced more rapidly than our ability to deliver them safely, effectively, and efficiently" (Institute of Medicine, 2001, p.25).

The demand for caregiving is increasing, with the chances of becoming a caregiver much higher today than ever before—and that likelihood will increase in the coming decades as the elderly population grows (Partnership for Solutions, 2004). Often these people need to devote many hours a week providing personal care and healthcare, and searching for resources for all the patient's needs. Further, they are facing a frequently confusing and uncoordinated array of services and healthcare arrangements. It is helpful for them to have a basic understanding of the variety of needs the patient may have.

What does all of this mean for you, the family caregivers, and for your parents? It means that as an illness progresses there will be increasing demands on you to address more care needs and interact with more providers in order to manage the illness and care between visits to doctors and hospitals. Patients and caregivers should be prepared to deal with a number of obstacles as they plot a course through healthcare and attempt to do it all on their own.

If you are a caregiver for someone with a serious chronic illness, or expect to be one in the foreseeable future, you can anticipate facing a number of critical issues, such as how to work with doctors' offices, hospitals, and health-related services. (For our purposes, family caregiving includes all unpaid services provided by family and friends.) Because of the gaps in healthcare and the problems with coordination, a great deal of what patients need between doctor's visits falls to such caregivers.

Your Parent's Doctor

It is important to know who your parent's primary treating physician is. Sometimes this is a doctor who has not known your parent over time. Primary-care doctors' offices are usually very busy, and most do not have the time, staff, or technology to help coordinate your parent's chronic illness or to help you fully understand all the treatment options. Efforts to create a "medical home" that coordinates care and provides ongoing health education and counseling are being developed by medical organizations. But with 80 million baby boomers reaching 63, the infrastructure for treating chronic illness is going to be severely challenged. Primary-care doctors are in great shortage: currently there are only about 100,000 family physicians and 100,000 internal medicine physicians in the United States, compared with over 700,000 specialists (American College of Physicians, 2006).

Keeping Your Parents Safe At Home—Wherever "Home" Is

As elder parents develop serious chronic illness, the specifics necessary to coordinate in order to keep them safe at home can become many and complex. Basic activities of daily living (ADLs)—eating, bathing, walking, dressing, using the bathroom—that were previously routine can gradually become difficult. Instrumental activities of daily living (IADLs)— housework, meal preparation, medication administering, shopping, getting to and from appointments, using the telephone, and managing finances—can also become harder over time. As frailty advances, many seniors begin thinking about moving, often from their home of many years, to senior living housing where various degrees of assistance are provided. There are different facilities to consider, depending on the person's degree of mobility.

As you will see several times throughout this book, a care-manager approach will help you understand the medical as well as nonmedical territory you are in and come up with a plan for coordinating your parent's care and finding credible in-home services to help them remain safe in their own houses. It is helpful to understand what options exist if, in time, staying at home becomes too difficult or simply not the best choice.

Independent Living: Independent living refers to facilities or residences within retirement communities for seniors who live alone and are fully functional (able to perform all ADLs). Residents in independent living have their own apartments or houses, although often shared recreational, social, and dining locations are also provided. The cost of independent living is about the same as buying a nice condo, with monthly expenses similar to condo fees.

Assisted Living: Assisted living refers to facilities that provide assistance and monitoring of residents to help ensure their health, safety, and well-being. These facilities provide care (such as giving medication and helping with bathing or dressing) for those who can no longer live alone but do not need 24-hour nursing-home care. Residents usually have their own private apartment, with access to on-site staff and common areas for socializing. Such facilities are licensed and regulated by each state, and may also be known as residential care homes, assisted care living facilities, or personal care homes. This can be relatively expensive—often about $4,000 to $6,000 a month.

Nursing Home: A nursing home, also known as a skilled nursing facility (SNF), skilled nursing unit (SNU), or rest home, is a facility for those in need of constant nursing care. People go to a nursing home when they can no longer perform many of the activities of daily living and need extensive assistance. Such facilities often provide ongoing assistance for elderly residents and may also offer rehabilitative services—especially in the case of accidents and reversible illness. Nursing-home care can be quite expensive, often costing thousands of dollars a month or more—although it may be covered by Medicaid or private long-term care insurance. Medicare covers nursing-home care only for beneficiaries who need skilled-nursing care or rehabilitation services following a hospitalization of at least three consecutive days. Such care requires a doctor's certification that it is needed.

Medicaid, on the other hand, covers ongoing nursing-home care, but only when the person has limited income and resources. Private insurance plans vary. Most elderly people, however, would rather stay in their homes, and there is an increasing array of private-pay services to facilitate this. A good care manager can help you and your parents decide what their particular needs are and to find credible local resources to help with private-duty, in-home care.

Family caregivers can be crucial in any one of these settings. Even in the best-run institutions, the needs of the residents can rarely be fully attended to.

The father of one of my friends was in a retirement home, and was quite comfortable. But because of his dementia, he frequently took long walks and forgot where he lived or how to get there. The director of the home told my friend and her brother that he would have to be put in a nursing home. They fought that, and then talked with some of the staff. One staffer suggested that they hire someone to stay with him during the day. She helped them find a part-time nurse and aide to help manage the care which the regular staff was too busy to attend to. The revised plan also had the treating physician adjust the dementia medications. With this help, my friend's father was able to stay in the retirement home until his death several months later.

Interestingly, there are examples of seniors who choose to move to what are called Naturally Occurring Retirement Communities (NORCs)—senior communities that have become retirement-oriented naturally, due to location or market forces, rather than by design.

Some of these innovative experiments in aging are building independent housing that allows each person or couple to own their own home but share a community plan for leisure activities as well as for medical and in-home care as aging and frailty advances or major illnesses occur. A care-manager approach helps look at the predictable needs of seniors and their family caregivers, helping to prevent a great deal of uncertainty and its resultant stress.

Over the next five years, there will be an increasing number of services and options that will allow seniors to "age in place," i.e., their home. Combining a care manager with a nurse or nurse practitioner who works with your parent's primary physician to carry out the daily, weekly, and monthly medications and ongoing doctor's office issues will be one option. There will also be more private-duty, in-home care (skilled aides) and telemonitoring (which can monitor your parent's blood pressure, intake of medicine, and movement around the house). This can help parents remain safe and independent at home for a longer period of time. In naturally occurring retirement community centers, where many seniors live in proximity, it is possible to deliver home support and services more economically.

Different Modes of Care

Hospital Care: Hospital admission usually happens for an acute-care event such as a heart attack, heart failure, difficulty breathing, stroke, serious infections, major injuries, or extreme weakness. Your parent may be admitted to an acute-care hospital via the emergency room or directly from a doctor's office. There are several types of acute-care hospitals—including academic medical centers (where teaching occurs with resident and intern doctors) and community-based hospitals. Many states have for-profit, as well as non-profit, hospitals (which include Catholic Healthcare hospitals) situated in most of their cities. It will be helpful to familiarize yourself with the hospitals in your parent's community. Hospitals often employ nurse care managers who help arrange the discharge planning. If a patient needs time to recover with more intensive nursing and physical therapy than is available at home, doctors will recommend 30 or more days in a rehabilitation hospital. Otherwise the patient is sent home.

Certified Home Care: Certified home care offers services covered by Medicare, commercial insurance, and Medicaid. These services are provided by home-care agencies certified by Centers for Medicare and Medicaid Services (CMS) and are available to homebound patients. Certified home care might include skilled-nursing care, physical therapy, occupational therapy, speech therapy, and home health aides. A doctor's order is necessary to obtain such services usually after a hospitalization or serious illness.

Private-Duty, In-Home Care: Private duty, sometimes called non-medical home care, refers to private services that include the work of home health aides, the provision of companions, and light housekeeping. Provided by home-care companies, such services are paid for by the patient or family, as Medicare benefits do not cover these services (except for the certified home-care services noted above). Some private and long-term care insurance, however, may cover the costs.

Hospice Care: Hospice is a comprehensive, family-centered approach to providing care for people in the terminal stage of an illness. It focuses on managing pain and symptoms, as well as providing physical, spiritual, and emotional support. Such services must be requested by a doctor, after the determination that the patient has a life expectancy of six months or less. These services may be part of a hospital or nursing home, but are usually provided in the home. (There are also hospice centers in which patients live out the last months of their lives.) Medicare covers most costs associated with hospice. In hospice settings, as well as in over 30 percent of hospitals nationwide, patients are treated with *palliative* care—medical care with the goal of relieving the pain, symptoms, and stress of an illness, rather than attempting curative care. Palliative care is typically provided by a hospital-based team that includes specially trained doctors, nurses, and social workers, in partnership with a patient's primary doctor.

How to Pay for Care

Medicare: Medicare is a government-funded social insurance program that supplies the elderly with health insurance. President Lyndon Baines Johnson signed it into law in 1965. Medicare is offered to all U.S. citizens and longtime legal residents who are 65 or older. In certain situations, younger people may also qualify for Medicare. In 2007, 43 million Americans were on Medicare. The baby boomers will all have reached 65 by 2031, so there will probably be 77 million Medicare recipients at that time. Medicare pays for 80 percent of covered medical and hospital services, and people who buy the program's

Medicare Supplemental Insurance have the other 20 percent paid for.

Medicaid: This is the U.S. health program for people and families with low incomes and few resources. It is jointly funded by the federal government and by individual states administering their own programs. It is the largest source of funding for medical and health-related services for people with limited income. It too was created in 1965.

Each state may have its own name for the program. Californians have Medi-Cal, while Tennessee has TennCare. Policies will vary from state to state, so if you are considering applying for Medicaid for your parent, be sure to find out what your state does and does not offer. Many elders qualify for both Medicare and Medicaid.

Long-Term Care Insurance: Private long-term care insurance helps pay for certain services to assist people who are too sick to perform ADL's like dressing, taking showers, or walking. The insurance also covers services within assisted-living facilities, adult day care, and nursing homes. These services are generally not covered by regular health insurance, Medicare, or Medicaid.

Managed Care: The term "managed care" can have one of several meanings. It is used to describe specific techniques to reduce the cost of providing health benefits while improving the quality of care, organizations that use those techniques, or systems of financing and getting the necessary care to enrollees.

According to the National Library of Medicine (1990), the term managed care encompasses programs "intended to reduce unnecessary health care costs through a variety of mechanisms, including: economic incentives for physicians and patients to select less costly forms of care; programs for reviewing the medical necessity of specific services; increased beneficiary cost sharing; controls on inpatient admissions and lengths of stay; the establishment of cost-sharing incentives for outpatient surgery; selective contracting with health care providers; and the intensive management of high-cost health care cases. The programs may be provided in a variety of settings, such as Health Maintenance Organizations and Preferred Provider Organizations."

Managed care provided by Medicare has limits on the services they provide. Some take the form of Medicare HMOs. Managed-care organizations often employ care managers to help control usage and costs. While this can be helpful, it's important to keep in mind that the primary interest of these care managers is the company they are working for. Their goal is to save expenses for their employers, not necessarily to do what is best for the individual patient. Care managers that you yourself hire to help you will work directly for you.

In 1973 the U.S. government passed the Health Maintenance Organization Act of 1973, which gave grants and loans to those wanting to start or expand HMOs. It also removed certain state restrictions for federally qualified HMOs. All employers with 25 or more employees had to offer federally certified HMO options alongside traditional insurance upon request (called the "dual choice provision"), though this provision expired in 1995.

This act also required HMOs to offer a specified list of benefits to all their members, to charge all members the same monthly premium, and to be nonprofit organizations. The act solidified the term "HMO" and gave HMOs increased access to employers. Not surprisingly, this caused HMOs to rapidly expand throughout the country. Meanwhile, the use of managed-care techniques also expanded, and such techniques are now found in a variety of private health-benefit programs. Ninety percent of Americans who have insurance are now in plans that incorporate some type of managed care.

Spouses of Ill Parents

Adult-children caregivers have to be concerned not only about the parent who is ill or frail, but also about that parent's spouse, who is also a family caregiver—and is usually the adult child's other parent.

Because the spouses of the senior patients are also family caregivers, they face many of the same care coordination, communication, and support issues noted above for the adult-children caregivers. In addition, such caregivers also cope with significant emotional and psychological burdens when caring for a spouse with a serious chronic illness. In the latest *Caregiving in the U.S.* survey by the National Alliance for Caregiving (NAC) and the American Association of Retired Persons (AARP) (2004), about 35 percent of family caregivers said taking care of the person they help was stressful. About a third also reported needing time for themselves. In addition, they needed help keeping their loved ones safe, managing their own emotional and physical stress, and balancing work and family responsibilities. All of these problems can take a toll on a caregiver's energy and health. This is especially true when a spouse's illness requires a lot of care and when it becomes more serious. Tension can also arise among caregivers: the spouse feeling that the adult children are discounting his role, the younger caregivers thinking they are more up-to-date and thus more efficient than the healthy parent.

One of the patients we provided with our care-delivery service was John Blackman. When his wife of 50 years was diagnosed with Alzheimer's disease, Mr. Blackman spent all of his time caring for her in their home. Mrs. Blackman was completely dependent on her husband for all aspects of her activities of daily living. He had to feed, bathe, and dress her each day, as well as do all the household chores. He had very little support from his children or other family members. Then he injured his back lifting Mrs. Blackman. Though his doctor told him he needed rest and physical therapy, he was unable to find the time. His injury persisted and eventually became debilitating enough that he needed back surgery. Only then did his children realize how bad things were going with their mother, and two of them moved into the house to take over the caregiving while their father had his surgery and time to convalesce.

Parents can conceal their evolving problems for many other reasons. They may fear that they'll be sent to a nursing home, or they may wish to save their children more anguish. A care manager can identify symptoms or problems that patients are avoiding and address them before they get worse.

Money Concerns

In addition to the stress and emotional issues you may face as a caregiver, you will probably also have to deal with a number of financial issues. Caregivers often miss work and lose income while looking after their parents. Depending on the family dynamics, it is helpful for the immediate family to make a financial plan for ill parents' needs. A care manager's help, which can solve complicated crises in as few as three to six hours, can cost up to a few thousand dollars a year if problems persist. However, the savings to families from investing in such help can reduce the number of long-distance trips that caregivers need to make, as well as their parents' hospitalizations and unnecessary treatments and tests, thus helping the families get the most out of their healthcare dollar. The private-pay nature of a nurse care manager can significantly improve the quality of care for those who can afford it, but to date leaves out poor and lower-middle-class families.

CSA, as we discussed in Chapter 1, was able to get funding for our studies from the public-health policy world, and we are hoping that, as the success of our program grows, that world will realize the efficiency (and, hopefully, the humanity) of such programs, and pay for care managers who work for families everywhere in the country. According to Arno, Levine, and Memmott (1999), the monetary value of family caregiving, if it were salaried, would greatly exceed the cost of outside long-term care services. A 1999 MetLife study found that on average, an individual caregiver loses $659,000 in wages, Social Security, and pension contributions because she takes time off or stops working. In addition, caregivers often pass up opportunities for training, promotion, and transfer assignments. Such costs can be even greater for long-distance caregivers who live less than three hours away—they spend an average of $386.00 per month on travel and out-of-pocket expenses. Those who live more than three hours away spend an average of $674.00 per month on travel and out-of-pocket expenses (MetLife, 2004).

One patient I worked with, Todd Green, had been hospitalized for kidney failure. One of his grown daughters lived nearby, while the other lived 800 miles away. Penelope, the daughter who lived in town, was the primary caregiver and spent a lot of time each day caring for his needs. Her sister, Jeannette, flew in one weekend a month to relieve Penelope. Jeannette spent over $1,000 a month on air fare, in addition to which she also had to use a vacation day each month to travel. When she was on the job, her work suffered.

This is not atypical. Total lost productivity for U.S. employers when their employees are taking care of older relatives is estimated at $33.6 billion a year (MetLife, 2006). In the future, then, employers would do well to put resources toward supporting caregivers, if not out of compassion, out of self-interest. A national Picker Institute study showed that 70 percent of medical consumers surveyed described the medical system as a "nightmare to navigate, impersonal, confusing, demeaning, and unresponsive" (Picker Institute, 2000).

Nowhere is the evidence for a care-manager approach to care coordination and health counseling greater than in the data found in Wennberg and Cooper's Dartmouth Atlas (Wennberg & Cooper, 1999). Looking across the country, Wennberg and Cooper discovered the disparity in effective medical care from state to state, and even city to city. Yet in some cases the availability of different procedures made no difference to the patient's health. For example, the Atlas clearly shows that patients in certain cities, such as Miami and New York, had more procedures and hospitalizations than patients in Minneapolis—yet the outcome was similar in terms of quality of care and longevity.

This research, as well as several other significant reviews of care in the United States, shows that more care is not always better care. Clearly consumers continue to need coordinating care (Fisher, et al., 2003a; Fisher, et al., 2003b).

Understanding Your Parent's Condition

In addition to the other services they provide, care managers help families be more discerning consumers of healthcare, thus enabling them to extract more value from their healthcare services and providers.

A care-manager approach will help you understand what questions to ask of all providers. Few doctors' offices have an electronic medical record that can transfer your parent's healthcare information to pharmacies, laboratory testing facilities, other physicians, home-care agencies, hospitals, and Medicare and other insurers. Gathering all the relevant information yourself is extremely time-consuming.

Sally Russell, one of the nurses on our staff, worked with an 82-year-old veteran with lung cancer. Like many veterans, Mr. Edwardson was proud of his stoicism and never mentioned his pain and discomfort to his children. When Sally came to work with him, she noticed that he winced from time to time. She asked if he needed painkillers.

"It hurts, all right," he admitted. But he refused the medication. When she asked why, he told her he wanted to wait until his pain increased. He feared that if he began using the medication when the pain was still bearable, he would build up a tolerance and it would no longer work when the pain became severe. Sally talked to his doctor, who told her that it wouldn't happen that way. Reassured, Mr. Edwardson began taking the pills.

These things happen frequently—and again, someone trained to recognize the signs is far more likely to pick up on what the patient needs than a harried and untrained caregiver.

What We Found Works

The eight activities that follow include the techniques that we have proven to work in helping family caregivers and their parents get the best care they can. Once you can identify the main problems that you and your parents are facing, you'll be able to create and follow an action plan. Many adult children, especially those who are long-distance caregivers, fear that their parents may have to move to assisted living or a nursing home because they are unable to care for themselves. That may or may not turn out to be the case. The specific details involved in your situation are the key: what exactly is going on, and how to figure out the details, come up with a plan, and make the best of the situation—even thrive while coordinating your ill parent's needs.

When the patient has Alzheimer's or other forms of dementia, a care manager can be especially helpful. The family caregivers usually have a larger number of tasks than most, and there is rarely the feeling of working *with,* rather than *for,* the patient. Their frustration can lead to anger—at the patient and at themselves for *being* angry. They know that the parent isn't deliberately being annoying, and yet they can't help feeling defensive and mistreated. The care manager is a good source of reassurance, conveying how common and unavoidable such feelings are, reassuring the caregiver that he isn't betraying the parent.

Of course, that feeling of betrayal isn't confined to caregivers whose parents have dementia. And sometimes these feelings can work against both patient and caregiver. Mark Nathan's widowed mother lived in Florida. Mark flew in from Chicago every two months. As her heart disease worsened, she became weaker and, at Mark's urging, moved in to an assisted-living facility. Mark saw this as temporary; he wanted his mother to move in with his family. But his wife and two teenage children didn't want this. For nine months the family argued about it.

Mark grew depressed, feeling that he had betrayed his mother by moving her from her home. On his next visit to his mother, he hired a care manager to help him look at the options and explore his guilt about his mother's situation. The care manager visited Mrs. Nathan to find out what she really wanted. When she told Mrs. Nathan about Mark's friction with his family, she was shocked. "Good heavens! I don't want to live there!" she exclaimed. "I love it here. I love living alone—and Chicago is *cold!*"

There are three main benefits to using a care manager that we have proven over the years. The first is that your parent will receive better care; the second is that it will improve the quality of life for both you and your parent, and the third is that it will improve the quality of the time you spend together. Whatever you and your parent discuss, plan, and do together in the time you are coordinating their care will leave you lasting and healing memories.

Over the years all of our care-manager programs, as well as our research programs, have shown that people often think of hiring a care manager only when a parent is already seriously ill. Sometimes, however, it makes sense to begin at an earlier stage, so that when and if the illness occurs, you'll be prepared. At the Center, we've had some good results with this.

One of the people who enrolled with our Your Support Nurse program was Cindy Lawrence, a vice president at a public relations firm. Her 81-year-old mother, Myrtle Herbert, had begun experiencing episodes of chest pain and shortness of breath and seemed to be slowing down.

Cindy anticipated that Mrs. Herbert would need her help as time progressed. She hired a care manager she had met in the course of her work. Fiona was warm, friendly, and highly experienced. The three of them talked frankly about Mrs. Herbert's age and health.

Fortunately Cindy and her family lived near Mrs. Herbert and the two had a strong relationship. Among other things, they wanted the care manager's help in finding a nearby assisted-living community before Mrs. Herbert needed it. If she never *did* need it, Cindy said, that would be great. The day after Cindy enrolled with us, she called Fiona. "I need your help," she said. Her mother had had a serious heart attack and was in the emergency room at the local hospital. The doctor treating her said she had to go to a teaching hospital right away and would probably need open-heart surgery. Cindy wanted to know about the hospital her mother would be sent to. Fiona assured her about the hospital, then helped her to write a list of questions for the doctor.

A care manager can improve care by knowing what to anticipate and by simply looking in on the home situation, assisted-living, or nursing-home conditions. She will know about community resources or benefits that are obvious only to a professional in the field. One of the nurses we trained was Doris Bowman. She was hired by Roger Nichols, a 78-year-old man who was the chief caregiver to his wife, Louise, a patient with Alzheimer's disease. She and Mr. Nichols moved to an assisted-living facility. After the move was made, Doris continued working with them. She saw how stressed Mr. Nichols had become, and suggested he might begin attending one of the many caregiver support groups offered by the Alzheimer's Association. But there were no support groups nearby, and he could not travel far from the home. Speaking later with one of the nurses at the home, Doris learned that there were a number of spouses there in Mr. Nichols' situation. Suddenly the solution came to her. They could create a support group right on the grounds of the assisted-living facility. The staffers at the home were enthusiastic, and soon they had a group going, right where it was needed most. As visitors to various patients learned of the group's existence, they too began to come to meetings. Though they didn't live at the facility, a loved one did, and to find the support group in the place that they visited was extremely helpful.

A care manager can improve the quality of life for family caregivers as well as their parents by helping to familiarize everyone with complex situations. First of all, an experienced care manager can normalize and explain an unclear situation to a first-time caregiver. Further, he can help caregivers gain control and efficacy around most situations.

Chapter 3 –
Physician Support and Health Literacy

Activity 1: Partnering with Your Parent's Doctors and the Doctors' Staffs

In coordinating your parent's chronic-illness needs with a care-manager approach, you will need accurate information and direction from your parent's primary-care doctor. This is the first step toward comprehending the specifics of your situation. You'll need to get a working understanding of your parent's diagnosis or diagnoses (many of the elderly have more than one condition). Simply knowing what these conditions are, and the relative severity of each, will help keep you more grounded and less powerless.

Once you have the diagnosis, you'll want to get the prognosis—the doctor's prediction of the illness's probable progress over a period of time. Your doctor may or may not volunteer this: don't hesitate to ask. Obviously the prognosis will depend on the particular disease. Further, it may change over time.

Early on in treating cancer, for example, the focus will probably be on a cure. If this doesn't happen and the cancer progresses, you'll want a new prognosis, this time focused on how the cancer can be contained. Again, this may take questioning. Not all conditions are easy to predict—advancing heart, lung, or kidney disease, for example. You can still, however, get the doctor's best estimate. Having a clear diagnosis and at least an indication of prognosis can be enormously helpful in planning caregiving routines. In CSA's care-manager approach to meeting parents' needs, the first questions our supervised nurse care managers, like many other care managers, ask are, "What did the doctor say your parent's physical problems are? What prognosis were you given?"

Once you have a diagnosis and prognosis, the next essential thing to know about is the treatment plan. Will it involve surgery, radiation, chemotherapy? Are there any routine outpatient procedures? What medications will your parent need, and how often? What are the side effects of the medications?

Family Involvement

In order to get the best information about diagnoses, prognoses, and treatment plans, you'll want to establish the role of various family members in communicating with your parent's doctors, the doctors' staffs, and all the treating providers. Within most families there is usually a primary caregiver, who assumes the responsibility of coordinating many aspects of the parent's care. Often this is the healthier spouse of the sick parent. Equally often, it is one of the adult children. It is important that all of you discuss who is to have this role, and what roles other family members (or involved close friends) will take on. There are numerous tasks for people to do, depending on where they live, what responsibilities they already have, and other individual factors. Who will be the one to contact other family members about the evolving situation? Who can commit to one-day-a-week caregiving in the home so the main caregiver can get some rest? The primary caregiver may (or may not) be the one who is going to communicate with the physician's staff and distribute information to the rest of the family. If not, you'll want to discuss which of the others can take on this role. This will prevent multiple and redundant efforts by various family members. It will also allow the chosen family member to create a working relationship with the doctor's staff. Once all this has been taken care of, the entire family can then implement the strategy that follows.

So achieving the best outcomes with ongoing serious illness depends upon coordinating physician expertise with what we call "an activated family unit." This unit involves the identified primary family caregiver(s), and an approach that can best be seen as partnering with your parent's doctors and the doctors' staffs. This "partnering" means that the involved family members depend on the designated family caregiver to get the information from the doctors and their staffs and relay it to everyone else, so the doctors aren't barraged with calls from family members. The primary caregiver will coordinate the information from multiple doctors' offices, integrate test results and treatment plans into the patient's and family's daily activities, and plan all of the home-based care that will be outlined throughout this book.

More and more doctors and their staffs are inviting these partnerships, recognizing that caring for elder parents is time-consuming and involves ever-increasing resources that the family members must provide. In order to best understand your parent's doctors and their staffs, it is helpful to recall the difference between acute and chronic illness, as discussed in the last chapter.

Studies have shown that patients rarely ask doctors questions and do not feel sufficiently knowledgeable about illnesses that they are coping with. Often, patients in their 70s, 80s, and 90s fear seeming impolite or are simply overwhelmed and do not speak up. For their part, doctors often feel rushed and do not have the time—or choose to have the time—to explain details of illness and treatment plans, especially when the patient does not seem to have any questions. Because the treatment can be complex, even if you or your parent gets the information from the doctor, you may still feel confused or bewildered about it.

Making the Partnership Work

A doctor's office can be an intimidating place from the moment you step into it. Much pressure can develop simply from being in a crowded waiting room. Further, interactions with staff members are often too brief to cover all you need to know. Doctors have a bad habit of standing rather than sitting when they discuss things with patients or caregivers, creating an aura of power—

they are literally looking down on you. Moreover, their conversations often seem rushed, and you may not have sufficient time to ask all the questions that are important to you. So you need to start with a determination not to be intimidated. Once you and your family develop a simple list of the questions that need to be asked, call the doctor's office and make an appointment to discuss the questions. Explain that it will take only a short time, but that it is essential.

When you meet with the doctor, get to the point as quickly as you can and convey your respect for his demanding schedule. For example, say something like, "Doctor, I have a few questions. I know how busy you are so I'll keep this as brief as possible." Most doctors will appreciate this and in turn respect your need for explication. The doctor may still resort to well-disguised exit strategies that are difficult for you to see. A common one is to refer you to reading materials you have been given. If possible, it would be good to have read these before the appointment, so you can say: "Yes, I read that and it was very helpful, but I still need to know about…" If you've just been given the materials, thank him and explain that you'll get to them right away, but for now you have certain pressing questions about your particular situation.

Typical questions are: "What is my father's working diagnosis? How can I understand what the diagnosis, prognosis, and treatment plan mean?" You might want to reframe this question based on the information the doctor has already given you: "Okay, you say my father has prostate cancer that has spread to his bones, and that the treatment plan is chemotherapy and radiation. Can you explain the pros and cons of those treatments, and how likely they are to cure him?"

Another response in keeping with the partnership approach is to initiate a form of "Teach Back" in which patients and families describe their understanding of a concept by illustrating the idea or bringing in a picture of the problem. For example, one of our CSA patients who suffered from advanced hearing problems drew his version of an ear canal and what he imagined was happening to cause his condition. The doctor instantly realized the extent of the patient's misunderstanding and how misinformed he was, and she reached for a medically illustrated chart in the exam room. "Let's use these illustrations—they're much clearer," she said. The chart gave the patient the information he needed, sparing himself and the doctor a time-consuming discussion.

One of the earliest indicators that you are developing a working partnership with your parent's doctor is that everyone will notice more satisfaction in the exchange. You will get the information you need and the doctor will realize that you are intelligent, willing to learn, and generally equipped to manage the problems without unnecessary follow-up calls. After all, in a successful partnership, both partners walk away contented with their work. If you feel you need help in assuming a partnership role, a care manager can help you, and even use tactics such as role playing to make you more comfortable and in control.

Once you have established a working partnership with the doctor, the telephone will play a large part in your work together. This may sometimes involve the doctor directly, and sometimes not. Often you will work with a specific nurse in the doctor's office. You can arrange an agreement with this nurse that you will be calling from time to time with appropriate questions based on a thought-out process.

One of the patients we worked with, John Kirk, had prostate cancer that had not spread. Every time he returned from his doctor's staff, his family would anxiously ask him what the doctor had said, and he would tersely reply, "Everything is okay." The family wanted to know more. Katlyn, the nurse care manager on his case, gave them a list of questions that they were to have Mr. Kirk ask the doctor. Paraphrased and adapted to the relevant situation, these questions can be used by most caregivers or patients. Making such a list is extremely important.

1. What is the prognosis? Is this a serious or mild form of cancer?

2. What are the treatment options?

3. What are the side effects of the treatment?

4. How quickly must the treatment be chosen?

After only several minutes with a nurse in his doctor's office, Mr. Kirk was able to get information that he had not known how to get in the two previous visits, and relay it to his children.

This particular list was a simple one, tailored to the patient's needs. Most of you will probably want a more detailed list, particularly if your parent's illness worsens. In addition to adapting the four questions above, here are some others you will probably desire to address:

- Can you cure the disease or is it going to get worse?

- Is the illness acute or chronic?

- What will it feel like if it gets worse and how can you help my parent be comfortable if it does?

- How will pain be treated? How will symptoms be treated?

- Can you speak a little more slowly so I can be sure I have it right?

- Can you put that in lay terms so that I can be sure I understand what you are saying about my mother's care?

- Do you have a picture that will help me get the idea?

- If I draw it out, I will remember it better and can explain it better to other family members. Can you help me do this?

- I thought I heard three different points in what you said. Can we go over each of them briefly one more time?

- Can I repeat to you what I heard so I can confirm that I have it right?

- I'm a bit embarrassed to say I don't understand what you are saying even though I know you explained it well. Can we go over it one more time?

In our experience doctors and their staffs can greatly benefit from having informed, prepared patients and families. An organized patient and family won't be confused, misinformed, or anxiously looking for services that they may not need.

This isn't going to be your last list of questions. You should do a lot of list-writing as more questions and more information come your way. Start by writing down everything you can get from your ill parent and whoever has been helping her up until now. Also get information from the doctors' staffs. Your parent will have to fill out permission for you to get the medical information, and then most doctors' staffs will have you speak with a nurse in the office for direct information. Not only does this allow you to review at a later date what the doctor has said to you or your family, but it also allows you to provide information to the doctor. For example, it is important to bring the doctor a current list of:

- All your parent's medications, current treatments, and tests

- The names and specialties of all other doctors your parent is seeing

- Questions for the doctor
- Any other family caregiver's questions.

Then whenever you take your parent to a doctor's visit, write a summary of the current situation. Keep in mind that most serious chronic illness cannot be cured, so it will probably progress, although it can stay stable for months and years. Questioning the doctor, then, will not be a one-time experience. When you anticipate the progression of serious chronic illness, you can plan ahead of time for how you will manage it.

Deal with Conflicting Opinions and Choose a Doctor You Can Trust

We have all heard about the value of getting a second opinion from another doctor, especially if you have any doubts about the treatment your own doctor suggests. This is a great idea, and it has reassured numerous patients when the original doctor's diagnosis or treatment recommendation has been echoed by another physician. It has also saved many people from unnecessary or incorrect procedures. But the downside is that very often two equally trustworthy and qualified doctors have conflicting opinions, so that you and your parent need to make a choice. Most people will ask their primary doctor, a family doctor, or an internist to help them if conflicting opinions between doctors arise. Usually it is helpful to have one doctor review multiple opinions and be certain that medications and treatment plans are understood and aligned.

Some disagreements among doctors have to do with which type of practice or hospital they are affiliated with, and what is available at different hospitals. Larger cities have academic teaching hospitals, where medical students, residents, and interns will be a part of the team you see, along with your attending physician. Some community hospitals have resident staff accompany the attending physician. So you will want to be clear about who is responsible for the case and who is taking care of your parent.

ACTIVITY 2: HEALTH LITERACY/UNDERSTANDING MEDICAL INFORMATION

In order to fully understand the medical needs of your ill parent, it's a good idea to further look at what is known as "health literacy." According to the Institute of Medicine, a person is considered to be health literate when he possesses the skill to understand information and services and can use them to make appropriate decisions about health (Institute of Medicine, 2004). Everyone, even healthcare professionals, can have difficulty with health literacy at some time or another. Medicine is a complex field, and there are new procedures, new diagnostic techniques, new medications, and even new diseases emerging all the time. Not everyone can know it all. Indeed, doctors and nurses themselves need continuing education, and to learn new medical information at different times. Yet patients and their caregivers often act as though such omniscience is their responsibility. How many times have you left your doctor's office knowing you did not fully understand what you were told about your health problems and what to do about them? Even when the doctor asks, "Do you understand?" or "Do you have any questions?" confused patients often answer, "Yes, I understand," or "No, I don't have questions." Today's seniors were raised in the era in which it was assumed that the doctor is always right. So they are likely to accept whatever she says even when they don't understand. When you begin helping them coordinate their care, you'll want to find out what they do and don't know about the ramifications of their condition. The care manager, who is a nurse or a social worker with experience in serious chronic illness and familiar with the complexities of medical information, can be an excellent guide in getting health-literacy information. As with any field, the medical profession speaks a language of its own that is useful when discussing cases with colleagues but often needs to be translated to laypeople. Be sure to learn as much of this language as you can.

Overcoming Embarrassment

One of the great hindrances to becoming health literate is embarrassment. People can feel ashamed to admit that they do not understand medical information that is presented to them. It isn't rational, but then, many feelings aren't. It is easy to revert back to old insecurities—to become once again the child in the classroom who hasn't done her homework and fears the teacher's scorn. But it's important to recognize and let go of such feelings—they get in the way of what you need to learn. To effectively work in partnership with your doctor you have to accept that medicine isn't your field of expertise but that you need now to become better educated about it. Once you recognize how much you can learn from questioning and from conscientiously listening to the doctor, you can begin to apply what you learn to your caregiving. This process can alleviate much of the feeling of inadequacy. None of your questions imply that you are asking too much of the doctor's time or that you are not paying attention to the details involved. Quite the contrary, our patients found that when they ask questions politely, pointedly, and with a therapeutic purpose, their doctors were quite willing to work with them.

Here is a typical story. John Nelson's father was ill, and John came to us to help him coordinate Mr. Nelson's care. He seemed very glum, and told the care manager, Rachel, that he was certain it was time to prepare for his father's death. Rachel asked why he was so sure of this. "Because when I rushed him to the hospital, they told me he had fluid in his lungs due to a weakened heart. That's always a death sentence, isn't it?" In fact, Rachel assured him, it wasn't. That diagnosis indicated congestive heart failure that caused fluid in the body to back up. It could be cleared within 24 hours with a simple diuretic. And though congestive heart failure was serious, this time it could easily be reversed without serious consequences. She gave him a website from the American Heart Association that explained the process.

Doctors are slowly coming to recognize the importance of using routine office visits to address the problem of health literacy. The American Medical Association Foundation has created a program for doctors entitled "Helping Your Patient Understand." Doctors are encouraged to speak slowly to patients, to use nonmedical language, to show patients pictures that clarify their condition, to teach in small pieces, to repeat what they say, to confirm understanding by asking patients to repeat back what they have learned, and to create a shame-free environment in which patients are encouraged to ask for clarification of anything they do not understand.

CSA studies have shown that doctors will spend more time with an activated patient or caregiver, and that the knowledgeable patient and caregiver will feel that they are getting more and better information than they have previously received.

Sometimes when a patient doesn't understand what the doctor says, there are particular reasons for it. If you can figure out what they are, it will help you get what you need to know. Here are a few likely reasons:

- Not knowing specific terms or words. Medical terms are always changing and can be very complicated. The trouble might simply be that you don't understand a word or term that was used. For example, if you don't know that a "fibroadinoma" is a benign breast lump, you won't understand that it isn't a cancer.

- Not understanding the context of the medical words being used. Even if you understand the overall meaning of a word (cancer, Alzheimer's, heart disease) or the names of specific lab tests, procedures (biopsy, chemotherapy, radiation therapy), or other services necessary, it may be hard to understand them in the context of how severe an illness may be, how far advanced it may be, or which form of a disease the patient may have (e.g., there are many different types of cancer and each type plays out differently and responds to different drugs).

- Having emotional concerns. Anxiety, fear, denial, embarrassment, and other emotional states can make it difficult to focus on the information you're being given.

- Having cultural differences. If you and/or your parent come from a different background than your doctor's, implications of some information may not be clear. Some doctors, for instance, come from a cultural background in which patients and their family members are not expected to understand the complexities of medical care. If this paternalistic "Doctor Knows Best" approach is part of the doctor's orientation, it will take more work from you to get the information necessary to make informed decisions. Sometimes cultural differences are not a question of nationality but of generation. The baby-boomer generation is much more of a consumer-oriented group than their parents and they expect more dialogue with a doctor.

- Having cognitive or functional impairment. Sometimes it is more difficult for a patient to read, write, speak, or even think if her own eyesight, hearing, or ability to think is impaired.

Daniel R. Tobin, M.D. with Karen Lindsey

Bringing a Family Caregiver Along to Important Visits

Even under the best of circumstances, health information can be confusing. When you are at the doctor's, there may be a number of things to remember, think about, and decide. Further, all the information that is being transferred can become anxiety provoking and emotional at times. Even if everything is presented in the clearest possible way, it might be hard to take it all in.

If you expect a particularly confusing or emotionally charged meeting between the doctor and your parent to occur, it would be especially useful for you, another family member, or a friend to go along. Take notes, and ask questions. In all of CSA's experiences over the years, we have seen this work wonderfully. At the end of the visit, the companion and the doctor can compare notes to make sure that everyone has the same understanding about what was said and what needs to be done.

One of the services that care managers can perform is to visit doctor's offices along with seniors and their adult children. In our work at CSA, it has sometimes been possible for our nurse care managers to speak with the nurse in charge of the doctor's office and obtain information that helps clarify diagnosis, prognosis, treatment plans, and health literacy—information that may be much harder for the patient or caregiver alone to get.

There are other ways to implement health literacy—books, articles, and of course the internet. These are discussed later in the book.

Remember, the first step in helping your parent is to understand the medical information about his condition. If you don't know something, always ask for an explanation, and keep asking until you're certain you've got it right. Doctors are not there to judge you; they are there to help you understand and to solve the problem of missing information.

Chapter 4 –
Information Support and Coordinating Care

Activity 3: Getting Information Support

Information support occurs when the care manager helps you learn how to gather and then use accurate health-related information. This is invaluable to caregivers and patients who need to manage chronic illness and cope with the stress it creates. Gathering information may sound easy, but it isn't. This chapter will show you how to do it well and efficiently.

Patients and their caregivers have wide-ranging needs that can be met when they have appropriate information. Often, families have to solve problems within complicated situations in unfamiliar territory, with multiple issues and many questions arising. While information support is involved in the medical arena, as we discussed in Chapter 3, that's only one area of need: chronic illness and its care involve legal, financial, emotional, and spiritual knowledge as well.

The need for information in so many areas can cause confusion and stress to both caregivers and patients. Studies have shown that patients who have greater informational support adapt better to surgery, experience less anxiety, require less pain management, and have shorter hospital stays than others (Krohne & Slangen, 2005). Essentially, the more appropriate information that a caregiver and patient have, the better they can cope and make good choices. In all of our experience at CSA, we have learned that information makes it easier for family caregivers and their parents to adapt to their new and evolving situation. Adapting requires understanding that the most productive way for both patients and caregivers to cope with the time ahead is to accept the new reality and to change with it. Ongoing informational support can be an essential component of helping parents be safe at home, since their caregivers have a wide understanding of all the ramifications of the illness and its progression. Before widespread use of the internet, accessing health information took more time and effort than it does now. The Web has changed all that. There is now much information available—sometimes too much.

Once you have obtained the information, the challenge becomes figuring out how to apply it accurately to your situation. How well you do this determines how useful it will be to you and your parent.

The accessibility of information brings its own problems. When thousands of facts are available at the push of a button, how can you determine which information is correct, and which is relevant to your situation? Americans today are facing a health-information overload: new studies constantly appear, often seeming to cancel each other out. Books, magazines, and television news reports add to the information glut. Therefore, caregivers and their parents have an ever-increasing need for reliable and concise sources of the *right* information. One of our clients placed her father in an assisted-living faculty she had found online, only to discover that the promised help with his daily medications wasn't forthcoming.

The problems with both overabundant and inaccurate health information can be addressed by having some guidelines when you start your search. It is important to be selective when gathering health information. Guidelines for deciding whether a book, magazine, or website is a good source of health information are listed below:

- The author or source of the content is established, respected, and dependable.

- The information is current and in keeping with current scientific findings and professional practice.

- The book or article is not focused only on selling a product and does not purport to have a turnkey solution to everything.

- The book or article is based on credible scientific research experience, identifies the source of its information, and provides references for the reader to access more information.

- The website does not charge a fee for information or membership.

- The website has limited advertising.

- The information provided is appropriate to the audience level and easy to use.

- The content is professional in appearance and tone.

- The content is not limited to one geographical location.

- The website has links to other sites.

There are advantages and disadvantages to gathering such health information by yourself. The positive side is that caregivers and patients are actively trying to gain control over dealing with advancing illness. Actively learning about chronic illness results in fewer misconceptions. Becoming comfortable with information can reduce anxiety caused by lack of knowledge.

The negative side is that if the family caregiver and patient become obsessed with the information, especially that obtained on the Web, their stress can skyrocket. A primary-care doctor that I have worked with over the years treats a number of chronically ill seniors. He found that many of them who spent hours on the internet thought that they had serious problems because of symptoms that turned out to be minor effects of their chronic illness. One patient came to his visit convinced that his ongoing headaches and advancing weakness indicated a rapidly spreading, incurable brain tumor. Fortunately, my colleague was able to reinterpret each symptom, and to send the man for a CAT scan, which showed that the symptoms were migraine-related and easily remedied with medication.

Caregivers can also experience this kind of stress secondhand, convinced that their beloved parent's disease is drastically spreading, based on ominous material online or in the newspapers. This phenomenon hasn't been studied, but it appears quite similar to what has been seen in medical students. Normally, these students showed themselves capable of interpreting information critically and intelligently. Then they began their initial course work in different categories of illness. Suddenly, many of them began to see parts of themselves and symptoms in the descriptions of illness they were studying (Hodges, 2004). This study shows that health-related information that is not confirmed or discussed with a professional can create unnecessary worry. Caregivers who have this tendency need to be aware of it and to guard against it. Push yourself into taking in information with a degree of detachment and a firm eye for context.

You should always check the information you gather with your parent's doctors before using it as a basis for any decisions. Professional care managers and certified home-care professionals (those who are paid by insurance or Medicare for 30 to 60 days) can always help you sort through information. If you are prone to rushing to judgment about health-related matters, you might time your reading and questions to coincide closely with your parent's next doctor's appointment, when the doctor or office staff can quickly place the information into context for you. Alternatively, you might ask the doctor to provide you with an individualized preface to any patient-education material that you plan to read, helping you rule out in advance anything that does not apply to your family's situation. At the very least, keep reminding yourself that worst-case scenarios don't always occur, and think instead about possible better outcomes. A friend of mine became so certain that her father's dementia would cause him to act out violently that she was certain he would hurt someone and, in a fit of remorse, kill himself. She told this to her brother, and added that if that happened, she would have to kill *her*self for not having prevented it. Her brother made her sit down, and firmly told her to be quiet. "So far, you've got everyone but me dead, so stop before you kill me off too!" He paused and said, "Okay, so that could all *possibly* happen. It could also *not* happen, and our job is to do everything we can to prevent it. Which is what we're doing!" He reminded her of the nurses' aides they were hiring to live with their parents, and the research they were doing into assisted-living facilities. In the end, predictably, no violence occurred and the situation played out as well as such a situation was able to.

This is not to suggest that you should stop looking for information altogether. There are good sources available and, as we've discussed, the more authentic information you get, the more control you can take of the situation. Many librarians at some community-based public libraries are receiving training in a new specialty known as Consumer Health Information Services. Some librarians will examine research in medical journals, review internet websites and health-related books, and prepare information packages for patrons. They will even mail the packet to a homebound patron. In at least one instance that came to our attention at CSA, a determined librarian located and contacted a health researcher to get an answer to a highly specific question. A similarly enthusiastic librarian linked a patron with a research study that provided participants with resources for preventing the common and devastating incidents of falls in the bathroom. In some cases, patrons can have question-and-answer sessions with librarians who are experienced in helping people find health-related information. For example, one library in New York arranged for the Office for the Aging to provide counseling assistance for seniors trying to understand the useful but complicated Medicare Part D benefits. Not all libraries have such dedicated personnel, but they do all have useful books and periodicals.

In addition to libraries, there are local and national nursing help lines that can be contacted free of charge to answer medical questions. Also, the National Association of Area Agencies on Aging provides free telephone referrals for specific community-based services that can help elders at home with transportation, Meals on Wheels, and crisis counseling. National disease-specific organizations such as the American Heart Association, the American Lung Association, and the American Cancer Society are often good sources of quality information support. The mission of these organizations is to provide information and education to family caregivers and patients. So what you get is usually up-to-date, reliable, and applicable to the illness in question.

For those family caregivers and parents who hire a care manager, this experienced professional should be able to quickly provide reliable informational support for health-related issues. No matter what the source of your health information is, taking an active role and asking questions will help you to gain a sense of control in the difficult situation you face.

Activity 4—coordinating Your Parent's Needs

As we noted earlier, one of the hardest things for caregivers to cope with is the many different sorts of issues that come up, each requiring different information from different sources. Coordinating all of these is a major task. A report by the Agency for Healthcare Research and Quality defined care coordination as "deliberate organization of patient care activities between two or more participants (including the patient) to facilitate the appropriate delivery of health care services. Organizing care involves marshalling of personal and other resources" (McDonald, et al., 2007, p.5). Care coordination involves pulling together multiple doctor's appointments, tests, procedures, medical information, home-care services, and as many other services as an adult patient requires to be safe.

For example, one family caregiver, Veronica Joseph, who was receiving professional care management services for her father, had significant long-term health problems of her own. She had received extensive and very expensive health care services, including surgery. Over time she was unable to keep up that part of the expense for which she was responsible. Because she was a proud person who had never been in serious debt before, she became increasing embarrassed as the number of invoices piled up and she began to receive incessant telephone calls from collection agencies. Worse yet, her health started to deteriorate and her need for care increased. The last phone contact she was able to tolerate with the healthcare provider was with the business office, which informed her that she would not be able to receive care in the future if she did not begin to pay her previous bills. It was especially troublesome because this health provider offered the particular specialty care that she needed for her relatively rare set of health problems.

During her previous discussions with Martha, the nurse care manager who was helping her with her father's illness, she had asked for help in information support. Several times she had asked Martha to research the internet and other information resources, and the care manager had found a large range of appropriate services for Mr. Joseph. Hence, Veronica was aware of how efficient an information search can be when performed by a professional.

Her discomfort about her health finances eventually spilled over into one of her consultations with Martha. When Martha understood how Veronica's embarrassment was causing her to avoid pursuing ways to resolve the problem, she offered to call the health provider for her. In this instance there were really two aspects to the information support Martha offered. One was obtaining information about the extent of the debt, for which particular services, and what the options were for paying for each type of service. Acquiring that information was easy enough because Martha had previously obtained the privacy permissions she needed. Further, she knew what questions to ask and how to help negotiate the best situation for Veronica.

The other aspect of this example of information support was what health professionals refer to as "advocacy services." Martha's profession made her comfortable interceding on Veronica's behalf. There are any number of situations in which a caregiver wants someone with "inside" knowledge to help deal with complicated problems relating to their own conditions. We will visit this notion of advocacy again later in Chapter 6. I bring it up now to make the point that in the care management process at one time or another any of the eight activities can overlap.

Few doctor's offices are set up to perform care-coordination services that link activities outside of the office setting. Many do coordinate medical care for their own services and try to integrate information from other healthcare providers. However, the link between the physician's office and other providers is seldom routinely coordinated with an electronic record. And at best, this will deal only with medical needs.

The pervasive lack of care coordination is well documented. A Partnership for Solutions review of chronic illness care coordination notes: "Many people with chronic conditions report receiving conflicting advice from different physicians and differing diagnoses for the same set of symptoms. Drug-to-drug interactions are common, sometimes resulting in unnecessary hospitalizations and even death. People with chronic conditions are getting services, but those services are not necessarily in synch with one another and they are not always the services needed to maintain health in functioning" (Partnership for Solutions, 2004, p.3).

The Institute of Medicine concluded in their review of chronic illness care coordination that "our current method of organizing and delivering care is unable to meet the expectation of patients and their families because the science and technologies involved in health care—the knowledge, skills, care interventions, devices and drugs—have advanced more rapidly than our ability to deliver them safely, effectively and efficiently" (Institute of Medicine, 2001, p.25).

There are several initiatives that are being developed throughout the country in which physicians are trying to improve care coordination. To date, however, this hasn't gone very far. If your parents are not in a managed Medicare plan or a demonstration study, they will not find a care coordinator or care manager within the medical-delivery structure to monitor and guide their ongoing needs. Currently the American College of Physicians (ACP) is conducting evaluations of a program known as the Advanced Medical Home. This program is described as a "patient-centered, physician-guided model of healthcare" in which staff in a doctor's office would coordinate patient care. The ACP proposes additional reimbursement for doctors to coordinate activities. This is a major step, but these services will not be available for quite some time. If your parent's doctor is part of a small practice with limited office staff, you are even less likely to find help with care coordination. Further, fewer physicians today are practicing primary-care medicine, turning instead to more lucrative specialties. In other words, a cardiologist, gastroenterologist, oncologist, and endocrinologist treating your parents are seen as specialty consultants rather than primary-care internists or family-practice doctors. Most parents will be working with their cancer or heart specialist for their primary information and may not be relying on their primary-care doctor for these conditions. Clearly, if a care manager were a part of the primary-care physician's office much of the difficulty family caregivers face would be greatly alleviated.

So, much of the coordinating will be up to you. Coordinating your parent's care competently will be at the foundation of gaining control over his well-being, as well as your own time and energy. But without training and expertise, it's a daunting job. A well-trained care manager, working within a company like CSA in which routine supervision is part of their ongoing education, is a professional, familiar with the complex but often predictable obstacles faced in the difficult stages of serious chronic advancing illness. She will bring together all the tasks needed for your parent's comfort—grocery shopping, lawyer appointments, medical scheduling, etc.

She can also guide you to resources and benefits that you may not know about, and she can help you to effectively communicate with busy health professionals. Like financial planners, college planners, wedding planners, and others, care managers fulfill an invaluable role.

But care managers still cost money, and not every family can afford to hire one. I've seen many instances of family members and patients who were able to figure out some of the basics of care coordination on their own. It is more difficult than having a care manager, but it can be done.

There is, for example, the case of Michael, a 52-year-old electrician who was devoted to his aging parents, both suffering from advancing heart disease and diabetes. They were growing increasingly frail, and he wondered if they needed to move to assisted living. Michael and his wife, Sarah, had three young daughters. They lived only 10 miles away from his parents, but taking care of their children and his parents became difficult. Adding to their distress was the fact that Michael and Sarah could not afford to hire a care manager or private-duty home care, so they dedicated several hours a night to searching the internet for information. Although it was not as detailed guidance as they could have gotten directly from a care manager, Michael and Sarah learned how to question the healthcare professionals taking care of his parents. They found that AARP had published a basic caregiving plan, which helped them to get started (See appendix for how to reach AARP). Their diligent work helped his parents manage their medications, prepare balanced meals, and keep up with the doctor's recommendations. All this cut back on Michael and Sarah's caregiving work, and enabled his parents to remain living at home for the foreseeable future.

Here are a few tips to consider if you take on the care-managing role.

1. Believe in your own observations and expertise. As you become involved with coordinating your parent's needs, you and your parent can learn the details of both the medical and nonmedical care involved. You will know every test that has been done, every medication that has been prescribed, and every treatment being undergone. Even if another relative or friend takes on part of the job (e.g., taking your parent to her doctor visits, cooking the family meals, etc.), you will know which person is doing which job at what time, and will get reports on any activities you are not directly involved with. Keep in mind that the family unit is uniquely suited to coordinate your parent's care once a working plan is organized based on the guidance and information that the family caregivers gather.

2. Stay organized. As we have noted earlier, medical care is fragmented and medical-service providers do not always have the time or ability to communicate with each other about your parent's care. You will probably see a number of health providers for different reasons. You may have a primary-care physician, several specialists, a nurse practitioner, home-care providers, pharmacists, and others. They are all looking at different aspects of the illness and may not communicate with one another.

Someone within the family should keep a record of all the services, tests, procedures, examinations, medications, and questions that need to be answered in order to coordinate care effectively. That person should keep an appointment book with enough space to write down essential information. At a minimum, you should have a record of:

- The names and contact information of each of your parent's doctors and other service providers (include a list of problems that each provider is addressing)

- Any tests, treatments, and procedures along with their dates

- A medication list

- Notes of past appointments with other providers specifically focused on the recommendations of each of these providers about treatments and follow-up

- A schedule with future appointments and the reasons for them.

Armed with this information, you should be able to tell each provider about all the medical care your parent is receiving from other physicians. Supply all the details—i.e., last week your mother saw her heart doctor, who increased her medication because she was having breathing problems. It is especially important to update all providers on any conditions that they may not be aware of—information you have included in your notes. Obviously if you are a long-distance family caregiver or otherwise unable to accompany your parents on their medical appointments, you will want to communicate with the physician's office as best you can. If possible, have a friend or relative who lives closer to your parent go along on doctor visits.

3. Keep everyone talking. In addition to your notes, make sure that copies of medical records, as well as any tests, treatments, or services, are forwarded to other providers who can benefit from the information you are coordinating. Keep all the providers informed about each other and be sure to ask each provider how you can best help keep medical tests and reports current. If you can identify a contact person at each provider's office, you will be able to follow up to make sure that everyone has all the important information.

In addition to sending and receiving information, getting to know the office staff in the doctors' offices can help you with planning and scheduling appointments. Often doctors' assistants keep cancellation lists to get patients in to see the doctor as soon as possible. If you take the time to talk with them, they may think of you first when the needs arise.

With good and well-coordinated information, caregivers and patients are better adapted and more in control of meeting the daily needs of living with an illness. The time spent finding the information, or the money spent hiring a care manager to help you, will save time later in the process—time which can be used to nurture both your parent and yourself and to enrich your relationship by creating room to express the intimacy between you—the one thing no one else can do.

Chapter 5 –
Guidance and Emotional Support

Activity 5—Getting Guidance Support for the Caregiver

Guidance support is the term used when a professional caregiver like a nurse care manager works with others to help them learn how to solve problems themselves, unlike tangible support, which occurs when the professional solves the problem for you. It is the cornerstone of CSA's approach. Care managers consistently provide guidance and information so that caregivers and patients can coordinate tasks and come up with action plans for solving problems. As we discussed in the last chapter, some people lack access to care managers, or the money to hire them, and need to become their own care managers. Though it's harder this way, it can be done. This chapter will outline some of the basic steps that guidance support involves.

As we noted in Chapter 4, it always helps to begin by creating a list of problems. The approach we discussed there is also used for practical, emotional, and spiritual activities.

Guidance support involves an uncomplicated problem-solving approach, and on reading about it you may feel that it is plain old common sense. And so it is. But it goes deeper than that: it involves a methodical use of "common sense" that siphons out components of self-deception, wishful thinking, or ignorance. This approach is adopted from long-standing therapeutic practices in the fields of both psychology and social work. The practical steps of guidance support involve learning how to identify family caregiving problems, gathering all of the facts possible in relation to the specific problem, coming up with an action plan that addresses those problems, and then checking to see if the plan is working. Problem solving with this care-manager approach will help you systematically identify and solve the most pressing problems that you face in addressing your parent's needs.

One of the jobs of a care manager is researching service providers in the community. In our experience at CSA, the more common nonmedical problems caregivers face involve helping parents stay safely at home rather than moving them to new housing, and understanding the finances of all the services needed as illness progresses. This includes the crucial distinction between insurance-covered services and private-pay services. Care managers can help design well-targeted strategies to gather all of the facts and create action plans.

Often, this care can involve emotionally charged issues within the family. Long-standing family conflict can become worse around advancing illness. Old clashes between parents and adult children that have lain dormant for years may come to the surface as illness and caregiver weariness provoke tension. Siblings too can relive old enmities as they argue over how best to help the ill parent or how to distribute caregiving responsibilities. One of the basic skills that are routinely demonstrated by care managers is working with family members to be sure that caregivers understand the exact nature of the problems they are facing and that everyone in the family listens closely for any differences in understanding or opinion, no matter how subtle. The care manager can lead family discussions, clarifying comments and asking leading questions. "Let me take a moment to be absolutely sure we're all on the same page," she might say. "In what I just summarized, did any of you understand anything differently?" When family conflict is old and bitter, the care manager can help access behavioral health specialists in the community.

It has been interesting at CSA to detect differences in understanding and opinion, even among family members who are very close. It is equally interesting, though saddening, to see how often adult children and their parents have been separated and estranged to varying degrees over the years. As parents experience advancing chronic illness, sometimes a sense of obligation may surface in the hearts of these alienated children—sometimes even a love that they never realized was there. When the parent has emotionally abandoned or even physically abused their children, there is often much anger and bitterness to deal with. Though these feelings can be painful to admit in the face of the parent's vulnerability, understanding them is necessary if the caregiving is to be helpful over a period of time.

Old family patterns—whether alliances or conflicts—have a way of tangling themselves around family problem solving. Often what families learn about their dynamics through a care manager helps not only with their current caregiving, but with the rest of their lives as well. Old wounds can be addressed and healed among siblings, who frequently recognize patterns that extend into their own parenting, and are thus able to make positive changes with their children.

One of the most pressing issues that arise for family caregivers is the question of helping parents to be safe in their homes. Advancing weakness due to Alzheimer's or other dementia, heart disease, advancing cancer, or general weakness can lead to a decreased ability to perform activities of daily living and can make it unsafe to continue living at home alone. Private-duty, in-home care can help, but a 24-hour, 7-day-a-week private-duty solution is too expensive for most people.

Another important area in which a care manager's skills are useful is anticipating obstacles that may emerge with any plan. A sense of urgency often results in caregivers rushing to enact a plan without thinking it through. Care managers often find that once a plan has been agreed on, it can be helpful to simply ask a few questions, such as "Have we missed anything that might help this plan work?" or "Our planning seems complete, but have we touched base with everyone who needs to know about it?" Such questions often jar caregivers into thinking about potential pitfalls they need to take into account.

Such questioning helped our client Mark August. He hired a care manager to help his parents, who lived far away, figure out how best to get them back to their old house after they had moved to an assisted-living facility. Neither Mrs. August nor her husband, who was battling advancing prostate cancer, were happy with their new living arrangements. Though Mark wanted to help his parents in person, there were too many problems and too many trips for him to make. Jenny, the nurse care manager, was able to talk with both parents and ask them the questions necessary to make this move possible. So helpful was she that Mark put her number in his mother's speed dial and told Mrs. August to call Jenny whenever she needed guidance. "She will help you ask the right next questions and show you accurate next steps," he assured her. Soon his parents were back at their old home.

Even after a plan has been put into action, its effectiveness needs frequent reviewing. A seemingly appropriate action plan may end up needing revision. One common difficulty for families is managing a parent's daily medication. Understanding the doctor's recommendations, arranging for medications to be picked up, and making certain that they are being taken regularly can sometimes require ingenuity. Even family caregivers who live near their parents can have difficulty with a parent who forgets or refuses to take medication as directed.

Obviously, this presents real dangers to the parent's health. One of our clients, Joanie Lamb, was her mother's primary caregiver. Mrs. Lamb had been on dialysis for 20 years, and now had end-stage renal disease. As she grew increasingly weak her doctor changed her medications, and she had to take 16 pills a day. One Sunday afternoon, Joanie left a week's worth of medication in the medicine cabinet, with a note that said, "Don't forget to take all of your medication." Mrs. Lamb, in her confusion, thought this meant she should take all the pills at once, and she did so. Luckily, she realized that she was becoming ill and called an ambulance. Her stomach was pumped in time to save her life. From then on, Joanie came by with a daily ration of medications. Joanie also contacted Your Support Nurse and hired a care manager. Penelope sat and talked with Joanie to work out a plan in which contingency helpers were enlisted to make sure that Mrs. Lamb took her medications correctly on mornings when Joanie couldn't get to the house.

The existence of private-duty, in-home services can help parents remain safe in their homes for a significant amount of time. It is important to periodically re-evaluate the number of services necessary and readjust the plan. Your parent's condition is likely to deteriorate over time, family dynamics can change in a number of ways, and the health professionals you work with may change jobs or retire. You need to be attuned to change and be ready to alter plans accordingly.

Private-duty, in-home care is becoming more prevalent throughout the country. It is wise to spend time choosing an agency rather than hiring someone whose credentials you don't know. Some private-duty agencies now work with care managers, beginning to integrate a nursing model that connects the seniors' home care with their doctors' treatment plans. This provides an excellent way to maintain your parent's independence and autonomy. Make sure to choose an agency that screens its aides and that keeps records of which aides work where, so that you can account for everyone working with your parent.

You should also know the difference between various kinds of people you are hiring. Does your parent need only companion care that involves light housekeeping, safety supervision, meal preparation, and medication reminders? Or personal care, that includes bathing and hygiene, feeding, help with transferring into and out of bed, and diabetic meal plans when needed? Finally, you might want skilled nursing, which involves wound care, feeding-tube assistance, and medical assistance such as colostomy needs. Working with the right agency and getting a sense of what your parent's needs are will get you the appropriate care.

There are examples of innovative care services arising in the country. A healthcare executive with an entrepreneurial spirit named Allen Hager has created an organization called Right at Home, a private-duty, in-home care franchise that sets standards for what a national service might look like. Right at Home companions and personal aides are carefully recruited, trained, and supervised. The organization utilizes innovative telephone mechanisms to maintain constant contact with patients and caregivers. Franchise owners are intensively trained, and home aides are respected and well compensated by industry standards in these franchises.

Another major area that guidance support can help you with is financial matters. Be sure that your parent's finances are well taken care of. Ask them about their money situation at a comfortable time, before financial problems arise. Many parents won't discuss this because it is an invasion of their privacy. Some prefer not to talk about money because they never want to be a financial burden to their children. Either the primary caregiver or another family member should commit to working with your parent to create and implement a financial plan. Issues such as financing healthcare, housing, and inheritance may be best facilitated in a family meeting or in individual conversations if there is no care manager to help. Financial planners and attorneys may initiate these conversations, but often these specific issues are avoided until crises develop. Seniors who have not thought out their finances are susceptible to fraud, and it makes sense for adult children to have financial conversations with their parents if the parents seem vulnerable.

Activity 6: Responding to Emotional Support

Over the years of working with people facing advancing illness, I have seen how varied and intense the emotions surrounding such illness can be for both the patient and the caregiver. I have also seen how little emotional support is afforded by healthcare professionals, who are absorbed in the physical aspects of healing.

Support for emotional reactions to advancing illness should be a part of routine healthcare. Some emotions manifest as clinical depression or anxiety, and when that happens they need to be addressed with psychotherapy and sometimes with medication. But worry, fear, anger, and confusion, as well as questions about self-worth and about the meaning of life are normal in the face of illness. They are predictable reactions—either from patient or caregiver.

Emotional Support for Parents

As chronic illness advances, parents will certainly experience a range of emotions brought on by illness and the fear of death. These emotions can contribute to a great deal of stress for the family caregivers. A good care-manager approach spends a significant amount of time focused on emotional support for the entire family.

Such support in the form of empathy from their healthcare professionals can help reassure patients as their disease progresses. But equally important is a larger, more complex response to emotions. Unpleasant feelings need to be addressed by loved ones, on a personal level, outside of the medical world. Even simply acknowledging and sympathizing with these emotions can be enormously helpful because it validates them.

We worked with one patient, a solitary widower of 83 with chronic heart failure. Mr. Charles told his cardiologist that he was becoming increasingly fearful about how much time he had left to live. Both of his parents had died in their 70s from similar heart problems. The doctor told him that his medications had been in existence for only a few years, and that it was much better than those that existed in his parents' time.

But somehow that wasn't helping Mr. Charles's anxiety. He had hired a care manager, and talked with her about it. She suggested that he bring it up again with the doctor, and also that he share his fears with his daughter. As he talked with both his daughter and the care manager, he realized what he was really afraid of. It wasn't so much about death itself: he was elderly, and knew his disease was serious. But he needed to talk about his fears of death and know that he was being listened to. He had been keeping his emotions to himself, and felt terribly isolated. Having the doctor, his daughter, and the care manager listen to him with concern and respect helped enormously to ease his fears.

Luckily, Mr. Charles was able to discuss his fears with his doctor, who offered sympathy and support. Many patients aren't. They conceal distressing feelings to avoid awkward interactions with providers and also to protect family members from more worry. Others simply want their doctors to concentrate on the illness itself and not spend precious time with nonmedical concerns. Feelings of shame can also play a part—abandoning the "stiff upper lip" can seem like weakness, even cowardice. Further, many physicians prefer to remain distant from their patients' emotions.

But worries and fears left unaddressed tend to add up and can harm a patient's health. Identifying anger and fear can help a caregiver in coordinating the parent's needs.

Emotional Support for the Family Caregiver

Most family caregivers experience a great deal of stress—specifically a form of stress that has been described as simultaneously objective and subjective. Objective stress is related to the amount of time and resources needed to care for parents, while subjective stress comes from the emotional burden that family caregiving can entail. Caregivers may feel that their parents are being too demanding and taking advantage of them. This stress can be intensified if they feel guilty for those emotions (Montgomery, Gonyea, & Hooyman, 1985).

One of the most helpful roles that a care manager can take on is to help family caregivers understand what the objective and subjective stress in caring for parents entails. Many primary caregivers are also taking care of their own children. Most are also holding down jobs—jobs that are now more difficult to perform, and also more essential in providing the finances needed for their other duties. Predictably, caregiver stress can lead to exhaustion.

Helping a parent with dementia can be especially difficult. One of our clients, Paula Evans, was helping her mother, whose Alzheimer's disease was slowly worsening. It was painful for Paula and her father when they realized that Mrs. Evans had difficulty recognizing them. For four months, they took care of Mrs. Evans at home, taking over cooking and household chores and making certain she never left the house without one of them accompanying her. This began to take an emotional toll on Paula and her father. Then they hired a care manager. Dale connected them with local support groups from the Alzheimer's Association. He helped them coordinate medical and nonmedical activities. He spent time talking with Paula, reassuring her that she was doing the best for both of her parents. He also helped both Paula and her father cope with the terrible pain of watching this woman they so loved puzzle over who they were. Paula began feeling less exhausted and better able to help her father care for his wife. And Paula now had more time to care for her own children and, importantly, herself.

What to Do

1. Be attentive—In order to address problematic emotions, you must first become aware of them. Pay attention to any changes in your feelings, physical and emotional. Are you more tired than usual—more than would be accounted for by the increased demands of your life? Do you feel constant worry? Are you less interested in the hobbies that you usually enjoy?

Equally important, note any changes in your parents' behaviors. Perhaps they sleep more or eat less. This can be a normal response to advancing illness, but it might be a sign of clinical depression, and should be heeded. They, even more than you, are likely to suffer from anxiety or depression over the drastic and incurable changes in their lives.

2. Stay connected—Support from extended family and friends can be a major help. They are likely to be aware of changes in your parent's behavior, as well as your own, offering another perspective that can help to spot problems. They can also help by providing respite from the routine chores of family caregiving. Having someone else cook, clean, or just sit and chat with your parent can give you a precious hour of solitude or recreation. They can also offer you a shoulder to cry on. People often ask if they can help when someone they know is going through

hard times, and they usually mean it. Don't be too proud to accept their offers.

3. Talk with the doctors—Once you notice that your parent is having an emotional problem, talk to the doctors about it. Addressing emotional needs is an integral part of complete medical care.

4. Seek additional help for yourself where needed—There are a number of sources of assistance for emotional issues, including support groups, counselors, and therapists. Support groups provide emotional sustenance for people experiencing similar life circumstances. Such groups are sometimes traditional meetings with a set time and place, or they can be large internet-based communities with members sharing stories via websites or e-mail. Usually credible groups can be found associated with hospitals or disease-specific organizations.

Always keep in mind that there is nothing "weak" about showing emotion. You are going through a highly intense experience, and highly intense experiences foster highly intense emotions. There is a wonderful medieval story about a young mother whose own mother is starving to death in prison. The younger woman is allowed to visit her mother, but may not bring her food or drink. The guards are all astounded that the old woman, who should be weak from hunger, is actually flourishing. Then they discover why: the daughter is breast feeding her mother, as her mother once breast fed her. So impressed are the authorities that they free the mother and her daughter, who becomes a town heroine.

What you are doing is the spiritual equivalent of the mythical daughter's nurturing: you are seeing to all the needs of the parent who once saw to all your needs. Never underestimate the depth of this decision—or of the emotions it evokes. It unites your past and your present, and it will profoundly enter your heart and help form your future. Allow yourself the myriad emotions this will evoke—and all the support you can get for those emotions.

Chapter 6 –
Tangible Support and Extended Planning

Activity 7: Obtaining Tangible Support for Your Parents

Serious chronic illness impacts all levels of a person's life. There are many practical needs and services that patients require as their illness progresses. Tangible support will be necessary over the days, weeks, and months ahead.

In addition to the services already outlined in this book, these practical services may include providing assistance with basic activities of daily living (ADLs; see Chapter 2). These include bathing, dressing, eating, using the toilet, walking, and getting in and out of bed. There are also the instrumental activities of daily living (IADLs), such as housework, meal preparation, medication administering, shopping, getting to and from appointments, using the telephone, and managing finances.

Family caregivers often attempt to address each of these needs when it arises. As the illness advances, the patient requires increased assistance. Inevitably, the sole caregiver soon becomes overwhelmed. Several efficient ways of arranging tangible support have been developed by many organizations, including Care Support of America.

If it's at all possible, you should avail yourself of some of these services. If not, you should try to find a way to get some help so you won't have to do everything by yourself. It is helpful to delegate a specific person for each service you require. Some of the support can come from family members and friends. Other services may require paid professionals. If the service is private-duty, in-home care, you'll want to have a contact at the agency. You'll also want to find out if there is any form of tangible support that can be obtained as a benefit from your parent's health insurance or as free services, which will cut back expenses. All of this can consume a lot of time and energy, and a care manager is invaluable. Once tangible support services are in place with reliable people and companies, much caregiver stress is relieved.

This becomes especially important for the caregiver whose parent lives far away. One of our clients, Michael Freeman, hired a nurse care manager from our service to help him arrange the care of his parents, who lived 800 miles away. Neither parent had a specific illness, but both were in their late 80s and slowing down. They were growing increasingly frail and weak, and it had become difficult for them to take care of their house. At first, Michael thought he could take care of everything himself. He contacted Meals on Wheels, a nonprofit agency that delivers meals to the elderly, and he hired a house cleaner.

But his parents were constantly phoning him for his help and advice, and he soon realized that every time he solved one problem, a new one arose. All this was taking him away from his work, which involved a great deal of business travel. One week Michael got a call from his mother's doctor, concerned because she was not taking her blood-pressure medications. That's when he called us. With our care manager's assistance, Michael was able to arrange private-duty, in-home care to help with routine shopping and ADLs. She was also able to help the entire family see that something needed to be changed. If the parents remained indefinitely at home, it was likely that eventually one or the other would end up needing to be placed in a nursing home. However, if they began right away to research assisted-living facilities and find one that both were comfortable with, they could apply and soon move there together. They did this, and continued to do extremely well with more assistance than Michael could have pieced together.

Monitoring

Sometimes fragile elderly people can remain living in their private homes with the help of a medical-alert device that can be worn and pressed to get quick help in an emergency. There are also more sophisticated home-monitoring systems that can report when your parents are getting out of bed and taking medications, though this can be too invasive for some people to tolerate. There are other, in-between services that provide regular phone calls to check for safety; to assess mental alertness; to make sure the senior is eating regularly and taking her medications, and to provide her with a brief social interaction. The frequency and timing of the phone calls can be based on the caregiver's request. Thus the caregiver can focus his phone calls on normal, pleasant conversation.

Some families are using monitoring devices that are connected to the telephone and can have the senior answer questions that the device is programmed to ask. Other telephone devices can even transmit blood pressure, breathing parameters, and weight gain for monitoring heart disease. New devices to better help seniors age well at home are being developed. Simple forms of home monitoring will transmit information to doctors and care managers as part of routine care. Emergency room visits and hospitalizations can be reduced with early monitoring and interventions, enhancing the peace of mind of caregivers and their parents.

Medication Management

It is very important to have a list of all of your parent's current medications, as well as a plan to be certain the medications are being taken at the proper time. Various methods of medication management are available. Tools such as day-of-the-week pill reminders may be all that is required. Frequently, though, something more involved is needed, such as equipment that measures the precise amount of insulin. There are also devices that monitor when medication is being taken. Other issues around medications can also come up—their costs, their side effects, the patient's ability to swallow them.

Transportation

There are transportation services designed to get seniors to medical appointments, ranging from private companies to community services geared to helping with these needs. Transportation may also be needed for other activities, such as shopping, getting a haircut, or going to the movies.

Family members, friends, and neighbors often provide transportation for seniors. Many cities have senior community centers that provide transportation to their activities. Public transportation can be used, either with or without a companion, depending on the nature and degree of the parent's illness. Some churches offer volunteer transportation services. If taxis will be required, get to know the cab company and its personnel, and establish yourself as a "regular." Just be sure you know who to call, and that person or organization's phone number.

One of the most difficult problems for seniors is accepting limitations on driving. You can get help in figuring out how to assess your parent's driving skills. There are checklists available (AARP website, Automobile Association of America website) as well as classes for tuning up driving skills.

Durable Medical Equipment

Medical equipment that is used repeatedly—such as wheelchairs, walkers, certain types of beds, movement aids, and glucometers for diabetes monitoring—are known as durable medical equipment (DME).

Anyone can buy this equipment, but Medicare will cover it only with a doctor's order. DME companies are accustomed to working directly with the physician's office to obtain the necessary paperwork. The company obtains medical information and makes certain that the doctor completes a Certificate of Medical Necessity (CMN). Medicare usually pays 80 percent of what they call "usual and reasonable cost."

A care manager can help if the patient is hospitalized, as the DME is often arranged by the discharge planner (see Chapter 5) and may be delivered to the patient's home before she is discharged. The care manager can also make sure someone is there to answer the door and oversee the transfer of the DMA into the house. If the patient is using a certified home-healthcare agency, that agency may arrange for DME. A care-manager approach suggests that the family choose a service using these criteria:

- Does the DME company service the patient's area?

- Since different companies specialize in different kinds of equipment, does the company you approach provide the kind you need?

- Is there a family preference for a particular company?

- Is this an established company?

- Does the company accept Medicare assignment— that is, will they agree to the Medicare definition of usual and reasonable, and charge the patient 20 percent of that?

It is important to know if your parent can drive to pick up equipment. The DME company should be familiar with requests to travel. For instance, if the patient uses oxygen and is planning to spend a month in a different state, the company can deliver travel oxygen and work with a DME company in the other state to deliver, set up, and service oxygen equipment.

Adult Day-Care Centers

Adult day-care centers are designed to provide care and companionship for seniors who need assistance or supervision during the day. Their programs free up some time for the caregivers, and provide seniors an opportunity to get out of the house and experience both mental and social stimulation. Not all states license and regulate adult day-care centers, and there may be great differences between individual centers. A care manager can give guidance and support about choosing an adult day-care program.

Costs vary among adult day-care centers, and they are not covered by Medicare. However some financial assistance may be available through federal or state programs, and the family should seek these out. Medicaid will pay most or all of the costs in licensed adult day-care centers and Alzheimer's-focused centers for participants with very low income and few assets.

Hospital Discharge Planning

Discharge planners are hospital employees, usually registered nurses or social workers, who interact with the patient, family, physicians, nursing staff, medical social workers, and case managers to assist with the post-hospital plans. The patient may return home with services to help secure safety, be placed in a physical rehabilitation setting for a short stay, or move to assisted living or a skilled nursing home. Not every hospitalized patient gets the services of a discharge planner, but every patient whose condition is serious can get access to one. Discharge planning may be recommended by the physician or nursing staff.

Financial Services

A financial planner is a person who assists others to plan for their monetary needs. Financial planners can have varied backgrounds. They can be licensed stockbrokers, accountants, tax attorneys, estate planners, elder-law attorneys, or money managers, in any combination. Anyone can claim to be a "financial planner." There is a certification specific to financial planners, but it is voluntary.

A financial planner can help identify a person's financial goals and offer strategies for realizing those goals. This planning is client-specific for different goals and different phases of life. A good plan will encompass all aspects that involve money and needs for future security. The goals can be long or short term, and may involve legal documents such as financial power of attorney (see below), wills, trusts, bank accounts, taxes, investments, and healthcare advance directives. Financial planners can also help with gathering information on legal issues and fraud, home repair and inspection fraud, Medicare fraud, and senior investment fraud. Some parents will not have planned their finances well or will have questions related to financing healthcare and other needs. Choosing financial planners wisely entails getting references as well as credible word-of-mouth recommendations. It is usually best to hire a certified financial planner (CFP), since the certification is regulated by the CFP Board of Standards, Inc., a reputable private organization.

Financial Power of Attorney

Also known as a power of attorney for finances, this is a document in which you give another person legal authority to act on your behalf concerning your finances. This person is called the *agent* or *attorney-in-fact*. You can create this document yourself, but you should consult a lawyer if you have reason to believe it may be contested.

Financial powers of attorney come in several different types. These documents can go into immediate effect, or can go into effect only when the signer has been certified as incapacitated by a doctor (known as a "springing" power of attorney). The documents can also give general legal authority to act on your behalf regarding finances, or be limited to specific financial situations, periods of time, or types of transactions (this is then known as a "limited" or "special" power of attorney). Finally, the financial power of attorney can be non-durable (it ceases to be in effect when the signer becomes incapacitated), or durable (it continues to stay in effect even when the signer becomes incapacitated). Most common financial powers of attorney are durable, so they can continue to have effect should the signer become incapacitated—and may be designated as springing or limited, depending on the specific situation and desires of the signer.

- The agent's job is to act on behalf of the client. An agent can have broad power to handle all types of personal finances. Or the power of attorney can be limited to specific items—i.e., paying the client's everyday expenses, running her business, investing her money, etc. The agent is required to act in the best interests of the client, maintain accurate records, keep the client's property separate from his own, and avoid conflicts of interest.

- Each state has different regulations and requirements for power-of-attorney designations. Caregivers, especially distant caregivers, should check on this to insure the validity of the document. There is usually a form that must be filled out completely and notarized. In some states, witnesses are required. This form may need to be filed with the local land records office. Legal advice from an attorney may not be necessary, but can be helpful to meet all state requirements. You may need to have your parent's doctor sign a statement verifying that the senior is of sound mind at the time of the signing. Some seniors may decide to make a videotape (this has the potential of working for or against the patient in verifying "sound mind.")

Where to Begin?

- You and your parent should gather important papers and make sure they are stored in a central location protected from fire or potential damage. (Some people like to give copies to a friend or relative, just to be doubly safe). The senior may want to have a Personal Information and Records Inventory List. This is a form that comprises an extensive record of pertinent information (unlike the medical list that focuses on health history). It includes but is not limited to the person's legal names and nicknames, address(es), phone numbers, and certificates: marriage, citizenship, passport, and birth, divorce, military service, etc. (This form can be obtained at www.agis.com.)

- You should have a discussion with your parent about her values, wants, and desires for now and the future. It's important that the caregiver and other family members understand how the senior thinks and feels, and to use that rather than their own wishes as the basis for any decisions.

- The financial impact of illness can be overwhelming. You can help your parent decide on the type of financial planner needed. Financial planning is an important part of preparing for the future. This impacts the caregiver as well as the care recipient. It is easier to be prepared when you know what you're facing. There are many financial and legal options available to help a caregiver to protect the parent's financial status.

There is also the opportunity for unscrupulous people to take advantage of this situation. It is important to know the credentials and experience of the financial planner being considered.

Protect against Fraud

- Check credentials. You're much safer with a certified financial planner.

- Do not sign papers until all requirements have been read and understood.

- Get a copy of signed papers at the time of signing.

- Keep records updated.

- If you need additional information, contact Certified Financial Planner Standards of Professional Conduct at 1-800-487-1497 or www.cfp.net.

When you have decided that you require outside assistance to help with a particular need of your parent, there are a number of issues to consider: What exactly do you need the service provider to deliver and does the company that you are evaluating provide this? For example, if you have decided that you would benefit from 20 hours a week of private-duty, in-home care, you may not need a nurse, simply a trained aide. Likewise, if you have decided that hospice home care is appropriate for your parent, you won't need to seek certified home care, but you will want the appropriate referral from your parent's doctor. If all you need is assistance with transportation, search for the best and most affordable transportation services in your parent's community rather than a more complex service.

ACTIVITY 8: DOING EXTENDED PLANNING

Extended planning is preparing for what can happen in your parent's foreseeable and long-range future. Few people do extended planning well. It is a difficult, often painful, process. We are used to searching for cures to medical problems, and we tend to focus on reversing disease and prolonging life. But in spite of all of the advances and technological breakthroughs of modern medicine, we remain mortal. Serious chronic illness leads in time to advancing chronic illness and to death. Facing this is essential to realistic extended planning, and thus to assuring that the remainder of your parent's life is as comfortable as possible.

The dynamics of extended planning involve everyone—the patient, the patient's spouse, and each of the children. Each needs to come to terms with the reality of the situation—and usually the reality is that the patient's illness will progress and end in death. In all the years that I have worked in health counseling and care coordination for patients and their loved ones, I have seen that it is usually the patient who first recognizes the approach of death. Family members each come to terms with this in their own ways and usually at different times. But the sooner everyone accepts the inevitability of advancing illness and speaks about it honestly, the more readily they can work on treatment plans that focus on physical and emotional comfort for the remainder of the patient's life, rather than on fantasies of cure or indefinite survival.

In some cultures, talking about advancing illness is thought to hasten it, and everyone involved needs to be sensitive to this. Care managers can find ways to facilitate culturally acceptable conversations about extended planning and prevention of avoidable crises.

You may be tempted to ask your doctor when your parent will die. But it is difficult for doctors to "prognosticate," as such predictions are called. Studies have shown limitations in doctors' ability to accurately prognosticate, with projections for each patient often being rough estimates (Christakis, 1999). (Prognostication should not be confused with "prognosis," which we discuss in Chapter 1. The doctor will usually know the typical course of a particular condition. What she can't do with certainty is tell you if a specific patient will die in three weeks or three months.) Rather than focusing on exact predictions, then, concentrate instead on adjusting to the progression of serious chronic illness, advanced illness, and dying. Doing this requires calmness and acceptance of the idea that there is opportunity for growth and closure in the last years, months, weeks, and days of life. It is possible with professional guidance to deal with advancing illness and end of life in a positive, pro-active manner. Beginning to explore these opportunities in the last years is often much more productive than suddenly initiating conversations when your parent is clearly in the last few weeks of life. It is helpful for you and your parents to look at extended planning together. This gives you all the opportunity to do some level of planning for what options will exist when the illness worsens.

One of our clients, Marlene O'Hara, initiated such a discussion with her 92-year-old mother. Mrs. O'Hara had advancing frailty, as well as heart and lung disease, and had moved to an assisted-living facility. Marlene attempted several times to talk with Mrs. O'Hara about what might happen if her heart disease progressed. At first, Mrs. O'Hara simply changed the subject. But on Marlene's third try, her mother looked at her and said, "Okay. I still plan to hit 100. But I can't live forever, so we'll talk about plans." This window of opportunity enabled the women to realistically plan for the future.

One of the most helpful conversation starters among families that I have seen used are questions such as "What preparations can we make now for when Mom's condition gets worse?" or "What can we expect to happen to Dad after this current treatment works?" When you have agreed upon a strategy, you can then bring up the topic with your parent.

Our CSA care managers have helped family caregivers by giving families questions that help facilitate conversations around extended planning. How should you initiate addressing the inevitability that advancing illness will move toward more suffering and less physical mobility? First, you need to give some thoughts to your own feelings about this. Then try to gauge your parent's comfort with the thought of the illness progressing. If she still maintains hope that she will recover, don't argue with her. She's moving toward acceptance at her own pace and with her own emotional tools. Instead, ask questions to see where she is in the process. "Where do you think your illness is going in the next several weeks or months? Are you afraid it might get worse?" If she says she thinks she'll either be cured or that her illness will stabilize, you can still address extended planning with a gentle "what if?" focus. First engage her in conversation about her future plans—if she says she'll be around for Cousin Joe's wedding next year, talk about how you'll go together. Then ease into the alternative possibility. "Great, that's Plan A, and it's a good plan. I think I'd feel more comfortable if we also had a backup plan, just in case we end up needing it." When you have gone as far as you can with that, wait awhile before addressing it. It doesn't hurt to make plans for Cousin Joe's wedding, and wishful thinking can sometimes be a great source of comfort. As the illness continues to worsen, you can again bring up extended-planning questions.

Additional structured conversations include encouraging the patient to think and then tell the family what she wants. "Any time my health problems get worse, I want to ask my doctor to coordinate how my symptoms will be treated. And if my illness continues getting worse, I want to ask about care that focuses on my comfort, in addition to all my other care." These two statements have been very helpful in looking at the fact that major illness of the elderly usually leads to situations that most of us do not discuss well at all. It is crucial to see what your parent responds to if you or a care manager involved in helping you coordinate her care poses the questions around extended planning. You need to approach the question of what may happen when the current illness worsens and to be able to hold the reality that serious chronic and advanced illness will eventually result in death.

It is not only family members who are uncomfortable initiating extended-planning conversations. Doctors, nurses, social workers, and even chaplains often evince the same discomfort. In our culture, dying has been seen as a disease that physicians fail to cure. So advanced illness and end-of-life conversations rarely happen within routine medical care.

Living Wills and Advance Directives

Over the last 20 years, one area of extended planning, at least, *has* been discussed a lot—living wills and advance directives. Familiarity with these concepts may be the key to motivate people to expand the conversation.

In a living will, the patient states what treatments he wants and does not want when he is no longer able to clarify this himself. It can be changed at any time before this occurs (if indeed it does occur).

Living wills are not legally recognized in many states, and they cover only some of the patient's concerns. The more universally accepted *advance directives* are documents that combine assigning someone (who must, of course, agree to accept the responsibility) to be a healthcare proxy with a provision that virtually constitutes a living will. This proxy is the only person who can make whatever decisions are necessary on the patient's behalf if he is unable to do so. If he doesn't have an advance directive or living will, it's a good idea for you to encourage him to make one.

Physicians rarely initiate conversations about living wills or advance directives, so patients and family caregivers will often need to seek out information on these tools. (For more information on advance directives, living wills, and healthcare proxies, see Chapter 5)

(If you yourself don't have an advance directive, now might be a good time to create one. Young, healthy people have been involved in sudden accidents, and there have been tragic cases of their dying without their wishes being honored.)

Pain Control

This is one of the largest areas of concern for people with advanced illness. Your parent is entitled to adequate pain management in all his care and treatments, and you may have to fight for him. Unfortunately, the medical world has not done an adequate job of educating and training doctors in the area of pain management, and Americans tend to be phobic about drugs. But the controlled use of opiates for pain control is a far cry from "recreational drugs," and your parent will not turn into a crazed drug addict. What *will* happen is that he will end his life with as little physical suffering as possible. If you are concerned about your parent's pain management, ask his doctor for a referral to one of the growing number of pain-management specialists (doctors or nurse practitioners).

The Spiritual Quest

In all my work with patients and family caregivers, I have been impressed that most people coping with serious illness ask age-old questions about meaning and purpose in life, and what role spirituality plays as they question their suffering and face mortality. Spirituality is not confined to a belief in a specific religion. Rather it is a connection to a force greater than oneself and one's thoughts and feelings. For some, spirituality involves a relationship to nature. Some see it as helping others. It may be perceived as a sense of connection to God, a sacred spirit, or a spiritual leader. Some believe in reincarnation and that the lessons of this life will shape their lives to come. And sometimes it is simply a deep acceptance of the traditional religion they grew up with.

In facing serious illness as a family caregiver or a patient, it is helpful to question what role, if any, examining a spiritual destiny plays in your life. It can be valuable to take a moment to reflect whether you feel that events in life are random or connected to a greater force.

The largest obstacle to facing the inevitable realities of dying is usually fear of death, a fear that our society has too thoroughly embraced. How does your parent view the next few weeks, months, or years, knowing that his disease will progress? How do the other members of the family view them? And how do *you* view them? Our staff has often worked with the patient's existential or spiritual beliefs. Studies have shown that, almost universally, we fear the dying process, seeing in it the loss of personhood. We fear being dead either because we believe that we will be punished for our wrongdoings in the next life, or we believe that after death we cease totally to exist. (I have known cases in which, paradoxically, the same person harbors both beliefs.)

In my own work over the years, I have seen a great difference between those who think they are going on to a better place (whether that is perceived as the traditional idea of heaven or something else) and those who think they are going into nothingness. Those who see a continuation of life beyond death experience significantly less fear or depression about dying than those who are convinced they will cease to exist. The idea of going to a better place or to be with loved ones who have died can bring about a sense of calm that mitigates much of the fear.

Often at this time, a patient begins to reexamine his beliefs about what life means, and what his life in particular has meant. Helping patients find such meaning has created some of the richest experiences that I have had in working with patients approaching the end of life. There appears to be a natural progression in the quest for interpersonal, emotional, and spiritual exploration, especially if the person is guided through a therapeutic process while illness advances. Even without a guide, however, it can be enormously helpful. We suggest that the patient ask himself questions such as:

- How can I live the rest of my life in the most meaningful way in terms of communicating with my loved ones? How can I best express my love for those people who are a part of my life, and apologize for any ways I've hurt them? And how should I tell them goodbye?

- How can I best reflect on my life and come to peace with the struggles I've had? How can I find meaning in the bad as well as the good aspects of my life?

- Who can I talk with about personal questions such as who I really am, where I came from, and where I might go after death?

One of the most moving experiences I have had with a patient came shortly after CSA began. I was introduced to Mark Adams by his daughter, Jamie. "He's 88 and he has advanced bone cancer," she told me. "He gambled away all our money when I was a kid, and messed up our lives pretty badly. I know he regrets it, but he can't say anything. I'm hoping we can have a family meeting to help him talk about this." As their care manager, I organized the meeting for them. It worked as well as Jamie had hoped. As we all started leaving the room, Mr. Adams said, "Dr. Tobin, can I talk to you for a moment?"

"Of course," I replied.

"I feel so much better being able to say I am sorry to my wife and kids for all the grief I created. I feel like I can now move on to wherever I have to go."

"Where is that?" I asked.

Smiling, he answered, "I'm not sure. But I *am* sure that I'm soul. It's not like I *have* a soul, I *am* soul, and I sense soul has to go to a next place. Soul comes here to learn lessons and I am ready to move on." He told me that he had developed a regular practice of daily contemplative prayer, during which he understood himself as "eternal soul."

Not everyone has such firm and intense convictions. Many people need to discuss and work through their beliefs about God, and what may or may not happen to the self after death. Sometimes people surprise themselves when they dig deeply within. Feelings and beliefs unexplored for years can reveal themselves—often joyfully, sometimes painfully.

Nor do all people believe in eternal life. But even the atheists I have worked with have wanted to wind up their lives by trying to understand what meaning or purpose they have had.

Most people, in my experience, do believe in some sort of God, and want now to think more about him and whether or not they'll be with him after death. Others see the eternal force not as a personal god, but as a larger, incomprehensible entity that they have come from and will go back to.

Our care managers always address this question with both the patient and the caregiver. It can be very useful to examine your own beliefs and those of your parent, and to see how those beliefs can best work together in helping your parent find the meaning his life has had.

Approaching the End

It can be hard for both the patient and caregiver to accept that the body will slow down. Sometimes before this happens, there is a sudden event, like a stroke or heart attack that causes death. Usually, however, advancing illness leads to a general weakness in which the person is confined to bed, and then breathing and circulation slow down and eventually stop. When you realize this, it becomes easier to view dying as peaceful, rather than as an emergency that calls for help. If your parent has not yet switched from treatment aimed at prolonging life to palliative treatment, he should probably do so now. Sometimes people have faith that God will provide a miracle at the last minute. If that is indeed the case, it will happen, whether or not treatment methods are changed. As your parent comes closer to the end of life, you will have to deal with the unpleasant decline of bodily functions. He will probably be incontinent, and you will have to deal with this. There is often extreme weight loss, making the patient look emaciated. Sometimes, if there is a lot of excess fluid in the body, it can create the opposite effect: he looks badly bloated. You, your family, and your parent need to be prepared for this.

As a death approaches, I have often seen the patient—and equally often the family members—embrace one of two extremes. On the one hand, there is the impulse to continue denying death with interventions such as feeding tubes, mechanical breathing machines, and antibiotics when the patient has pneumonia. All of these are sensible tools while there is real possibility of cure, but they all too often keep the patient alive in pain, and for only a brief time. If it's what your parent truly wants, you should accept the decision. Otherwise, listen carefully and accept it when your parent chooses to accept dying and to let it happen unhindered.

At the opposite end is the controversial question of suicide. I think it's a bad idea; and certainly any patient considering this should think deeply and long before going through with it. I have found very few patients who decide to end their own lives, once they have been reassured that they will be given effective pain relief. If this is something your parent considers, you yourself will need to think about it, dig deeply into your own soul, and find your own beliefs. You also need to look at one very practical fact. Assisting suicide may be moral or immoral, mentally healthy or unhealthy. But in this country, it is unambiguously illegal.

Between the extremes of invasive interventions and suicide is the acceptance of death, with palliative care to see the patient through the process. I once heard of a European doctor who said to an American colleague, "You Americans act like death is optional." It isn't, but there *are* options in how we approach death and dying, and those are the ones we need finally to come to terms with.

Taking care of your parent from illness to end of life can be painful, terrifying, and heartbreaking. It is also one of the greatest things you can do in your life. Again and again, I have seen amazing growth occur within this process—even for those whose relationships with their parents have been strained or distant. Watching this, I have come to believe that we are hard-wired to care for our aging parents much as parents seem hard-wired to care for their young children. I sense that the meaning we find in caring for our parents helps to shape the opportunities that will exist for caring for ourselves as we grow old. A care-manager method of parent care contains the basic person-centered, humanistic approach that can guide public policy toward supporting and sustaining the vital and profoundly civilized work of family caregivers.

Appendix –
Resources for Caregivers

General Caregiving Websites

AARP Caregiving Websites
The home page with articles, access to tools, and featured online groups.
www.aarp.org/family/caregiving/

A chart of long-term care costs, such as home health aides, throughout the United States.
www.aarp.org/family/caregiving/articles/state-by-state_long-term.html

General information about Medicare, state-specific coverage, links to related sites, coverage for long-term care, home health care, and convalescent care.
www.aarp.org/health/medicare/medicare_interactive_counselor.html

Online communities on AARP.org: There are 11 groups on caregiving topics as well as groups on grief and loss,

Alzheimer's, cancer support, heart disease, and many others.
www.aarp.org/community/groups/

Eldercare Locator
This site or call center is a good place to start when you are looking for help in a local community. It will provide information on local resources and contact information for state and local agencies.
www.eldercarelocator.gov

Family Caregiver Alliance
The FCA is the first nonprofit in the United States to support caregivers with information and advocacy.
www.caregiver.org

Lotsa Helping Hands
A site useful for organizing friends and family to support care.
www.Lotsahelpinghands.com

National Alliance for Caregiving
Provides resources, planning guides, research reports, and policy papers for caregivers.
www.caregiving.org

National Association of Area Agencies on Aging
Coordinates the network of local Area Agencies on Aging. Contains information, as well as locations and contact information for the local agencies.
www.n4a.org

National Family Caregivers Association
Provides excellent information for caregivers.
www.nfcacares.org or www.familycaregiving101.org

Strength for Caring
An online resource and community for family caregivers that helps them take care of their loved ones and themselves.
www.strengthforcaring.com

Care Manager Websites

The National Academy of Certified Care Managers
Maintains credentialing and certification for care managers.
www.naccm.net

The National Association of Professional Geriatric Care Managers
Provides information on geriatric care management.
www.caremanager.org

Housing and Homecare Websites

American Association of Homes and Services for the Aging
Represents primarily not-for-profit organizations.
www.aahsa.org

Medicare.gov
Provides a guide to judging the quality of care provided in nursing homes across the country.
www.medicare.gov/NHCompare

National Association for Home Care and Hospice
Site contains information and an agency locator.
www.nahc.org/

National Citizen's Coalition for Nursing Home Reform
Provides information for consumers on long-term care and contact information for state agencies.
www.nccnhr.org

National Private Duty Association
Site contains information for caregivers and patients on home care, as well as resources to find local home-care providers.
www.privatedutyhomecare.org

Visiting Nurses Associations of America
Provides home health information and a list of local Visiting Nurses Associations.
www.vnaa.org

Respite Websites

Faith in Action
Interfaith volunteer caregiving program of the Robert Wood Johnson Foundation.
www.fiavolunteers.org

Hospice and Palliative Care

Hospice Foundation of America
Contains hospice locator and information on hospice care.
www.hospicefoundation.org

National Hospice and Palliative Care Organization
Information about end-of-life care.
www.nhpco.org

Training

American Red Cross
The American Red Cross has developed how-to programs for family caregivers. Check with your local Red Cross for classes in your area.
www.redcross.org

References

American College of Physicians. (2006). *The Advanced Medical Home: A patient-centered, physician-guided model of health care.* Philadelphia: American College of Physicians.

Arno, P. S., Levine, C., & Memmott, M. M. (1999). The economic value of informal caregiving. *Health Affairs, 18,* 182-188.

Christakis, N. (1999). *Death foretold: Prophecy and prognosis in medical care.* Chicago: University of Chicago Press.

Fisher, E. S., Wennberg, D. E., Stukel, T. A., Gottlieb, D. J., Lucas, F. L., & Pinder, E. L. (2003a). The implications of regional variations in Medicare spending, part 1: The content, quality, and accessibility of care. *Annals of Internal Medicine, 138,* 273-287.

Fisher, E. S., Wennberg, D. E., Stukel, T. A., Gottlieb, D. J., Lucas, F. L., & Pinder, E. L. (2003b). The implications of regional variations in Medicare spending, part 2: Health outcomes and satisfaction with care. *Annals of Internal Medicine, 138*, 288-298.

Hodges, B. (2004). Medical student bodies and the pedagogy of self-reflection, self-assessment, and self-regulation. *Journal of Curriculum Theorizing, 20*, 41-51.

Institute of Medicine. (1997). *Approaching death: Improving care at the end of life*. Washington, DC: National Academy Press.

Institute of Medicine. (2001). *Crossing the quality chasm: A new health system for the 21st century*. Washington, DC: National Academy Press.

Institute of Medicne. (2004). *Health literacy: A prescription to end confusion*. Washington, DC: National Academy Press.

Krohne, H. W., & Slangen, K. E. (2005). The influence of social support on adaptation to surgery. *Health Psychology, 24*, 101-105.

Mathematica Policy Research, Inc. (2001). *National public engagement campaign on chronic illness: Physician survey*. Baltimore, MD: Johns Hopkins University.

McDonald, K. M., Sundaram, V., Bravata, D. M., Lewis, R., Lin, N., Kraft, S. A., et al. (2007). Volume 7: Care coordination. In K. G. Shojania, K. M. McDonald, R. M. Wachter, & D. K. Owens, (Eds.), *Closing the quality gap: A critical analysis of quality improvement strategies: Technical review 9*. Rockville, MD: Agency for Healthcare Research and Quality.

MetLife Mature Market Institute. (1999). *The MetLife juggling act study: Balancing caregiving with work and the costs involved*. Westport, CT: Metropolitan Life Insurance Company.

MetLife Mature Market Institute. (2004). *Miles away: The MetLife study of long-distance caregiving*. Westport, CT: Metropolitan Life Insurance Company.

MetLife Mature Market Institute. (2006). *The MetLife caregiving cost study: Productivity losses to U.S. business*. Westport, CT: Metropolitan Life Insurance Company.

Montgomery, R. J. V., Gonyea, J. G., & Hooyman, N. R. (1985). Caregiving and the experience of subjective and objective burden. *Family Relations, 34*, 19-26.

National Alliance for Caregiving & AARP (2004). *Caregiving in the U.S.* Washington, DC: National Alliance for Caregiving.

National Library of Medicine (1990). *Medical subject headings (MeSH)*. Bethesda, MD: National Library of Medicine.

Partnership for Solutions. (2004). *Chronic Conditions: Making the case for ongoing care*. Baltimore, MD: Johns Hopkins University.

Picker Institute. (2000). *Eye on patients: A report by the Picker Institute for the American Hospital Association.* Boston, MA: Picker Institute.

Tobin, D. (2000). *Peaceful dying: The step-by-step guide to preserving your dignity, your choice, and your inner peace at the end of life.* Cambridge: Da Capo Press.

Wennberg, J. E., & Cooper, M. (Eds.). (1999). *The quality of medical care in the United States: A report on the Medicare program: The Dartmouth atlas of health care 1999.* Chicago, IL: AHA Press.

About Your Support Nurse

Your Support Nurse (YSN) is a proven and practical national nurse care-manager service provided by Care Support of America that helps family caregivers identify, coordinate, and solve the needs of aging parents. YSN has been shown to improve the quality of life for family caregivers and patients.

For more information, visit:
www.YourSupportNurse.com
www.CareSupportOfAmerica.com

About the Authors:

Daniel R. Tobin, M.D., is a nationally recognized leader in advanced illness health counseling and care coordination. He is the author of *Peaceful Dying* and coauthor with Joanne Hilden, M.D., of *Shelter from the Storm*. Dr. Tobin is the founder and CEO of Care Support of America and serves as Adjunct Assistant Professor of Psychiatry (Health Psychology) at Dartmouth Medical School.

Karen Lindsey is the coauthor of *Dr. Susan Love's Breast Book*, *Dr. Susan Love's Menopause Book*, *Peaceful Dying* (with Daniel R. Tobin, M.D.), and *Shelter from the Storm* (with Daniel R. Tobin, M.D., and Joanne Hilden, M.D.). She is also author of *Divorced, Beheaded, Survived* and of two books of poetry. She teaches writing, literature, and women's studies at Emerson College and the University of Massachusetts in Boston.

Printed in the United States
125945LV00001B/1-201/P